AN EXERCISE IN UNCERTAINTY

AN EXERCISE IN UNCERTAINTY

*A Memoir of
Illness and Hope*

JONATHAN GLUCK

HARMONY
NEW YORK

Harmony Books
An imprint of Random House
A division of Penguin Random House LLC
1745 Broadway, New York, NY 10019
harmonybooks.com | randomhousebooks.com
penguinrandomhouse.com

Library of Congress Cataloging-in-Publication Data
Names: Gluck, Jonathan author
Title: An exercise in uncertainty / by Jonathan Gluck.
Description: First edition. | New York: Harmony, [2025] |
Includes bibliographical references.
Identifiers: LCCN 2025000863 (print) | LCCN 2025000864 (ebook) |
ISBN 9780593735787 hardcover acid-free paper | ISBN 9780593735794 ebook
Subjects: LCSH: Gluck, Jonathan | Multiple myeloma—Patients—United
States—Biography | Cancer—Patients—United States—Biography | Cancer—
Treatment—Psychological aspects | Uncertainty—Psychological aspects
Classification: LCC RC280.B6 G587 2025 (print) | LCC RC280.B6 (ebook) |
DDC 616.99/418—dc23/eng/20250414
LC record available at https://lccn.loc.gov/2025000863
LC ebook record available at https://lccn.loc.gov/2025000864

Printed in the United States of America on acid-free paper

2 4 6 8 9 7 5 3 1

First Edition

Book design by Diane Hobbing

The authorized representative in the EU for product safety and compliance is
Penguin Random House Ireland, Morrison Chambers, 32 Nassau Street,
Dublin D02 YH68, Ireland. https://eu-contact.penguin.ie

To my parents, Eugene and Elizabeth Gluck
To my sisters and brother, Jennifer Gluck, Bettina Henderson, and Andrew Gluck
To Dr. Lon Weiner, Dr. Steven Gruenstein, Dr. Paul Richardson, Dr. Sundar Jagannath, and Dr. Shambavi Richard
To anyone whose life has been touched by illness

Above all, to Didi, A.J., and Oscar

Contents

Author's Note

This is a work of nonfiction. The people and events depicted in it are real. In one instance, I changed the name of a fellow patient I met in the hospital to protect her privacy. (I've noted as much in the text.) In two other cases, I changed the identifying details of an individual to protect their privacy for professional reasons. All other names and details are real.

This book has been thoroughly fact-checked, particularly with respect to medical and scientific information. To be sure I remembered events correctly, I consulted a second source whenever possible to confirm my recollections.

A portion of the proceeds from this book will be donated to multiple myeloma research.

PART ONE

The Slip

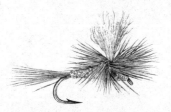

1.

IT WAS ONE of those lousy late-fall New York evenings, cold and dark and sort of half raining and half sleeting. I walked out of my office and slipped on a patch of ice. It wasn't much of a slip. I just twisted my left hip, then caught my balance. I went on my way. This was in November 2002.

The next morning, my hip hurt. I've had sports injuries over the years, and it felt like that—a torn ligament, maybe. I figured I'd rest it and it would go away. Then a few weeks went by and then another few weeks, and it still hurt. In January, I went to see my orthopedist. He took X-rays but didn't see anything wrong.

My hip kept hurting, but I didn't go back to the doctor. I was thirty-seven years old and healthy. A sore hip didn't seem important.

2.

BEFORE I SLIPPED on the ice that night, my life was about as good as I could have hoped for, maybe better.

My wife, Didi, and I had gotten married five years earlier. We had met in 1993 in San Francisco, where we were both starting our careers as journalists. For a short time, we worked at the same magazine. I thought Didi was cute, smart, and funny, and she later said she thought the same about me, but we were both seeing other people. After a few months, Didi moved on to a new job.

About a year and a half later, Didi and I ran into each other at a mutual friend's party. My previous relationship had ended, and Didi's, she let on, was teetering. We had a good time talking, and as we were saying good night, I mentioned that it might be nice to get together again sometime. The next day, we had lunch. That night, we went to dinner and saw a movie. Later that week, Didi broke up with her boyfriend, and she and I began dating.

Didi is tall and thin, with brown hair and a warm, welcoming smile. She is strong, determined, independent, and preternaturally energetic. She is passionate and unguarded; what you see is what you get. She can be serious and goofy, sometimes in the same sentence. She has more friends than anyone else I know. Although Didi was born and raised in the United States, her mother and father are from Buenos Aires and Berlin, respectively. She speaks fluent Spanish and loves to travel. She also loves music, everything from opera and musical theater to eighties alternative rock. I defy you to name a Smiths or Simple Minds song she does not know. She has a strong interest in fashion and beauty, with a charming high-low personal style. No one pairs an H&M sundress with a Saint Laurent bag more attractively. She and I share a sarcastic sense of humor. We like many of the same books and movies. We both swear a lot.

Not long after we started dating, Didi and I fell into a ritual of having coffee and bananas together every morning for breakfast. At a ceramics class she took, she made me a mug and saucer with a message painted on it: A PERFECT UNION. COFFEE AND BANANAS . . . AND YOU AND ME. I shared the sentiment.

One of the first things Didi and I bonded over when we started dating was that we were tired of San Francisco. We missed our families back east, we missed the change of seasons, and San Francisco offered limited opportunities for journalists.

We decided to move to New York.

In our early days living in the city, Didi and I led the kind of life many young people starting out in New York hope to lead. We had good jobs. We made new friends. We went to concerts, museums, and plays. We ordered cheap take-out food and haunted late-night dive bars. We had our favorite pizza place, bagel shop, and neighborhood pub. If we complained about our bosses, the smell of the subway platforms in the summer, and how high our rent was, it was all part of the adventure. Our apartment, a studio on East Twelfth Street in Greenwich Village, wasn't really big enough for the two of us, but we made it work. For a time, we stored one of my suitcases in the oven.

In May 1997, I proposed to Didi on top of the Empire State Building. It was supposed to be a surprise, only I didn't count on the security checkpoint on the way to the observation deck. Didi was kind enough to pretend she didn't see me take a little blue box with a silk ribbon tied around it out of my jacket pocket and stash it in my backpack before I sent the bag through the scanner and passed through the metal detector. A few minutes later, looking north toward Central Park, I asked Didi to marry me, and she said yes. A pair of German tourists were the first people to know we were engaged.

That fall, Didi and I got married in Amherst, Massachusetts, a picturesque New England college town. I had gotten my undergraduate degree there, and Didi, in what we took as a sign, had grown up there. I was thirty-two, Didi was twenty-six.

A month or so before our wedding, the rabbi asked us each what we loved most about the other; then during the ceremony she told the congregation what we had said. Didi said she loved that I always considered other people's perspectives, that I was thoughtful. I said I loved that Didi was "real." I meant that she isn't afraid to see things as they are, that she doesn't shy away from problems.

3.

THAT WAS MY personal life. I was also doing well professionally. In San Francisco, I had started out as a fact-checker at a parenting magazine and worked my way up to senior editor level. After I moved to New York, I worked at *Men's Journal* magazine, editing long-form feature stories about everything from ill-fated mountaineering expeditions to environmental disasters and eventually serving as deputy editor. I had a close-knit group of colleagues there. We worked hard and stayed out late. We were like college friends but with paychecks.

In July 2000, I took a job as the cofounder and editor in chief of a startup magazine for young lawyers and law students. Launching a publication from scratch is one of the most challenging and exciting things you can do in the magazine business. I was fortunate enough to land several well-known contributors, and the publication went on to be nominated for a National Magazine Award, the industry's highest honor, in its first year of eligibility.

On the night the other editors and I finished the inaugural issue and shipped it to the printer, I walked home through Washington Square Park. It was almost midnight, but the park was full of people. A busker played "All Along the Watchtower." Couples sat around the park's iconic fountain holding hands. The lights of the Empire State Building, visible uptown, worked their magic. I had grown up in a small former mill town in upstate New York. For years, I had dreamed of coming to New York City, but the truth was that

I wasn't sure I could succeed there. As I walked through the park that night, I felt like I maybe kind of sort of had. I let out an embarrassing little yelp of joy.

As East Coasters, urbanites, and Jews, Didi and I felt at home in New York. Because both sets of our parents had lived in the city as young couples, it felt like we had come full circle. Even after 9/11—in fact, especially because of it—we felt a deep connection to New York. In July 2002, with help from my parents with the down payment, we bought an apartment not far from the one we had been renting. We wanted to make the city our permanent home.

About a month after we moved in, I was doing the dishes one night when I heard a scream from the bathroom. It was Didi. Because this was New York, I assumed she had seen a cockroach. Didi came running into the kitchen. She was holding a telltale plastic stick.

4.

THE FOLLOWING FEBRUARY, I heard about a job opening at *New York* magazine. A pioneer of what's called the New Journalism, a blend of nonfiction reporting and novelistic storytelling techniques made famous by writers such as Tom Wolfe, Gloria Steinem, and Nora Ephron, *New York* is considered one of the best publications in the business. I enjoyed my job at the legal magazine startup, but the opportunity was too good to pass up, and I wound up getting an offer. I worked with an amazing team of writers and editors and published stories about everything from childhood sexual abuse in the Orthodox Jewish community to the expanding role of food carts on the New York culinary scene. It was a dream job.

Still, it was only the second-best thing that happened to

me that year. On April 29, 2003, our daughter, Abigail Juliana, or A.J. as we call her, was born.

For the next few months, Didi and I rode the crazy train of exhaustion, confusion, and elation that is new parenthood. Three A.M. feedings were administered. Anxious calls were placed to the pediatrician. Bedtime stories were read. Baths were given. Silly songs were sung. From her earliest days, A.J. liked to stroke the hair on my forearm as she fell asleep. When she was old enough to talk, she called it "petting my fuzzy arm."

What can I tell you that you haven't already heard from other new parents? That A.J. was adorable? That Didi and I were smitten? That she was our everything? All of those things were as true as the truth gets.

5.

THAT FALL, IN November, I realized a full year had passed since I had slipped on the ice. Not only had my hip not gotten better, but it had gotten worse. It hurt all the time. I couldn't run. I felt a stab of pain whenever I coughed or sneezed. It was getting hard to pick up A.J. *It's been a year since I did this,* I remember thinking. *It's not going away on its own.* I went back to my orthopedist, Dr. Lon Weiner, who ordered an MRI.

I remember worrying about getting claustrophobic in the machine; that was what I considered a major medical issue. But after I had the MRI, I basically forgot about it. Worst case, I thought, I might need surgery. A day or two went by, and I got a call at work: "Dr. Weiner wants to see you. He's got your MRI results."

This is how naive I was: I thought, *Wow, that's great. This guy is calling me with my test results before I even have a chance to call him.* Five days after the MRI, I went back to Dr. Weiner's office. The receptionist took me straight to an examining room.

One of the things about growing up in the television age is that we've seen all of the big acts of the human drama—weddings, births, deaths—played out before we've experienced them. What happened next had an eerie feeling of familiarity about it.

Dr. Weiner came in and closed the door. He sat directly across from me, fixed me with a professional gaze, and said, "I've got the results of your MRI. There's a lesion on your hip." Only this wasn't *ER,* and Dr. Weiner's voice, dispassionate as he tried to make it, contained an unmistakable trace of actual human horror.

"A lesion?" I said. "You mean a tumor?"

"Yes," he said.

I was thirty-eight years old, married to a woman I loved, working in the job I had long wanted, and living in the city I had dreamed about living in since I was a kid, in a lovely new apartment. I was the first-time father of a seven-month-old daughter.

And with that single syllable, I had cancer.

6.

AT THE TIME I learned I was sick, I was told I had between eighteen months and three years to live. Thanks to revolutionary treatments for my illness, many of which have been developed only in the time since I was diagnosed, that was more than twenty years ago. It is not a stretch to say I am a medical miracle.

I'm also part of a new and rapidly growing group of people. In recent years, researchers have developed novel therapies that have transformed not just multiple myeloma, the rare and incurable bone marrow malignancy it turned out I have, but many other cancers from a death sentence, with a period at the end of it, into a chronic illness that many patients live with for years, if not decades, an ongoing story, final chapter unwritten.

Nationally, the overall cancer mortality rate fell by a third between 1991 and 2019, according to the American Cancer Society, and the pace of that decline has accelerated from about 1 percent per year during the 1990s to 1.5 percent per year during the 2000s and to 2 percent per year from 2015 through 2020. That means more people are surviving the disease and going on to live their lives, many of them for prolonged periods.

To be clear, when I talk about people living with cancer for significant lengths of time, I'm not only referring to people who have been cured of the disease; I'm also talking about people like me who live with incurable but treatable cancers for many years, often undergoing one difficult, if not debilitating, therapy after another to keep us going, treatment by treatment. Those of us in this group could be said to make up a new kind of zombie race, one that isn't damned to be forever half dead and half alive but rather permanently half sick and half well. We are cancer zombies.

And it's not just cancer. Researchers are developing breakthrough treatments for illnesses such as multiple sclerosis and sickle cell anemia that are helping patients who suffer from those conditions live longer despite not being cured.

At the same time, long-term illness in general is becoming more common. According to a National Health Council report called *About Chronic Diseases,* "generally incurable and ongoing chronic diseases," such as heart disease, COPD (chronic obstructive pulmonary disease), rheumatoid arthritis, and diabetes, afflict some 133 million Americans, or more than 40 percent of the U.S. population. By 2020, according to the report, that number was projected to grow to some 157 million. About half of all adults have a chronic health condition, and approximately 8 percent of children ages five to seventeen are said by their parents to have one or more chronic diseases or disabilities. Almost a third of the population is living with not just one chronic illness but two or more conditions, according to the NHC, and that number is rising. In 2009, chronic diseases accounted for 70 percent of deaths in the United States, the National Research Council says, with heart disease, cancer, and stroke accounting for more than half of all deaths each year.

7.

WHAT'S IT LIKE to live with an incurable illness for more than twenty years? How has it affected me? My wife and children? My family and friends? My career? My finances? What's it like to live with the knowledge not just that my disease might come back but that it *will* come back, only I don't know when? How do I deal with the anxiety that brings? The fear? The uncertainty? What's it like to live in a state of perpetual uncertainty?

This story is my attempt to answer those questions, to draw a detailed map of this new and largely uncharted territory of human existence. In sharing my experience, I want to show people living with long-term illnesses, those who love and care for them, and anyone else, for that matter, what that landscape looks like. I want to illustrate not only that it's increasingly possible to survive a serious diagnosis longer than ever before but also that it's possible to have a successful career, raise a family, enjoy the company of friends, and pursue hobbies and interests you love while living with an incurable long-term disease. That outcome is by no means guaranteed—some ten million people worldwide still die from cancer alone every year—but today, more than at any other time in history, it is a realistic hope. I am living proof.

As I will note more than once in these pages, cancer has very little good to offer. But living with a near-constant awareness of my mortality for more than two decades has also taught me valuable lessons about how to live. At least I hope it has. I aim to share that knowledge, too.

In one sense, my story is unusual. As increasingly common as it is, serious long-term illness is still, fortunately, the exception, not the rule. But in another way, my story is universal. At some point in life, who doesn't confront adversity? Who doesn't experience fear and anxiety? Whether it's a frightening medical diagnosis, the climate crisis, war, job loss, the covid pandemic, or simply the difficulties of everyday life, who doesn't face uncertainty?

Cancer, as I would come to learn again and again, is an exercise in uncertainty. But then, so is life.

PART TWO

Diagnosis

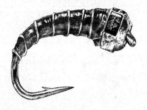

1.

WHEN YOU FIRST learn you have cancer, you don't think about the next twenty years. You think about the next twenty seconds.

In my case, my first reaction was denial. "No. No, no, no, no," I said to Dr. Weiner. "This isn't possible. I'm thirty-eight years old. I feel fine." And then: "I have a seven-month-old daughter. This cannot be true."

I used to think of denial as a pop-psychology cliché. Not anymore. Denial is a vital human coping mechanism. It helps cushion life's inevitable blows.

Dr. Weiner showed me the MRI report. The key portion read: "Large osseous lesion (9 mm × 7 mm × 4 mm) on left hip. A large probable lytic lesion involving the left acetabulum extending to the left ischial ramus. Differential considerations include a primary osseous malignancy such as chondrosarcoma, although a metastatic lesion should also be considered. Further evaluation with a whole body scan is recommended."

Deciphering medical jargon is a critical part of learning how to navigate any serious diagnosis, and my crash course in that language started right there in Dr. Weiner's examining room.

"What is 'osseous'?" I asked.

Bone-related, Dr. Weiner said.

"What about 'lytic'?"

The destruction of bone due to a disease.

"Acetabulum? Ischial ramus?"

Portions of the socket part of the ball and socket that is your hip joint.

"Chondrosarcoma?"

Bone cancer.

"Metastatic lesion?"

A tumor caused by one cancer that spreads to other areas.

"What is the difference between a tumor and a lesion?"

A lesion refers to any area of damaged tissue. A tumor is a specific type of lesion. All tumors are lesions, but not all lesions are tumors.

That last answer seemed to provide a bit of hope. Maybe my lesion wasn't a tumor, after all. I started tossing out crackpot theories and terms I don't really know the meaning of. Could the lesion be some kind of calcification or bone spur? Dr. Weiner said it wasn't likely.

The tumor was in a tricky spot, he said. He said I'd probably need chemotherapy, as well as surgery to remove a large portion of my pelvic bone. The best-case scenario, he said, was that he could fuse my hip afterward, using a cadaver bone, and create a sort of semiprosthetic leg. Another possibility, something he implied but was kind enough not to share with me at the time, was that he would have to amputate my left leg. His euphemism was that I might be looking at "a much more extensive disability."

Dr. Weiner's office is on the twelfth floor of Lenox Hill Hospital, overlooking East Seventy-seventh Street. Across the way, a group of children were playing on a rooftop playground. I remember watching them and thinking, *My daughter will never know her father.* Unlike denial, it's not clear to me what evolutionary purpose self-pity serves at a time of crisis, but that was what I felt.

The first person I called, oddly enough, was my boss. I was suddenly, urgently, concerned about being late for work. I initially thought the feeling had something to do with being responsible, but I see it now for what it was: a way to delay telling the people closest to me what was going on.

The next person I called was my therapist, Dr. Barbara Gol, a psychologist and psychoanalyst whom I'd been seeing for roughly five years. She occupied the sweet spot that a therapist occupies in your life: She knew me well, but from a certain distance, and she had the training and experience to handle a situation like this. I trusted her. She agreed to see me right away.

As I stood on the downtown 6 train platform, images of surgeries and chemotherapy began flooding my thoughts. I wasn't suicidal, but it occurred to me that New York, with its skyscrapers, bridges, and subways, offers the incurable cancer patient any number of helpful methods for checking out, an unsung virtue of the greatest city in the world.

2.

WHEN DIDI IS happy, she's happy. When she's sad, she's sad. When she's angry, she's angry. All that unchecked emoting is one of her most lovable qualities. But in this case, it made me afraid that she might flip out.

Dr. Gol and I talked for some time; she got me settled down. Then she asked me if I'd like to tell Didi right there, now, in her office. It seemed like a good idea. I called Didi and asked her to come meet me.

When she arrived, about a half hour later, she had that look on her face that people have when they know their life is about to change. As best I can recall, this is what I said: "I have some bad news. I got the results of my MRI this morning, and there's a tumor on my hip. They're not sure what it is yet, but the thing they want me to do is have more tests as soon as possible so they can figure that out. I asked them if it's possible it's nothing, and they are pretty certain it's not nothing."

Didi didn't flip. She barely said anything. She cried briefly, then just took my hand and held it. I didn't know it then—in our six years of marriage to that point, Didi and I had never faced anything this upsetting—but that's how Didi reacts when something awful happens.

Didi's mother and father, Estela and Julian Olevsky, met in Buenos Aires in the summer of 1965. Julian, a violinist, had emigrated with his family from Germany in 1935 to escape the rise of Nazism, when he was nine years old. Estela, a pianist, was born in Buenos Aires; her grandmother had come to Argentina from Italy, and her father had come from Austria.

That summer, when Julian was playing a concert and looking for an assisting artist, his manager introduced him to Estela. He was thirty-eight, she was twenty. The first piece they played together was called *The Devil's Trill Sonata* by Giuseppe Tartini. The first time they played it, Estela says, she knew they were a match.

Julian and Estela fell in love, began playing concerts together around the world, and eventually settled in Amherst, concertizing and working as music professors at the University of Massachusetts. In 1970, Didi was born.

On the night of May 25, 1985, at around 2:00 A.M., Julian had a heart attack. Didi was asleep, and Estela went to the hospital without her (an uncle happened to be staying with them).

Didi woke up early the next morning when Estela came into her bedroom, red-faced from crying. "Is it Daddy?" Didi asked. Julian had a history of heart disease.

"Yes," Estela said.

"Is he dead?"

"Yes."

Julian was fifty-nine years old, and Estela was forty-one. Didi was fourteen.

Because Didi wasn't old enough to cope with the loss of a parent, she basically swallowed her feelings about it. Now that's her reflex whenever something particularly upsetting happens. That tendency would prove to be problematic for both of us, but at that moment in Dr. Gol's office, when I had all the emotional upset I could handle, a calm response was just what I needed.

That night, I gave A.J. her bath, read her a story, and put her to bed. I stood by her crib for a moment. What I remember thinking is *Yes, the universe contains a death force, and that force is closer to me than it's ever been. But there is also a life force. I need to believe in the life force.*

<h1 style="text-align:center">3.</h1>

I HAVE NO meaningful family history of cancer. I don't smoke. I exercise and eat reasonably well, and drink moderately. So what made me sick?

My main theory was 9/11. I lived and worked in downtown Manhattan at the time of the terrorist attacks on the World Trade Center and for years afterward. Despite claims to the contrary from officials, who later apologized for their statements, the air, as we now know, was far from safe. In fact, it contained high levels of toxic chemicals, including benzene, a substance used to make jet fuel, exposure to which is a known risk factor for multiple myeloma and other cancers. On the other hand, I also learned that most experts didn't believe at the time that such cancers would show up so quickly. I once asked one of my doctors about this, and his answer was "Who cares?" He wasn't being flip; he was being philosophical. Since I can't go back in time, why worry about it?

Other theories that have cycled through my mind at 3:00 A.M.: I used to carry my cellphone in my front pocket, next to my left hip. My family used to tease me about eating an excess of orange foods—Cheetos, Doritos, Gatorade—while I was growing up. Did the water in my hometown contain carcinogens? My mother used to tell stories about how the runoff from the carpet mills would turn the water in the local Chuctanunda Creek yellow. Maybe I should have been nicer to people. Karma.

Despite not being religious, I found myself praying. For some reason, it was important to me to pray alone and secretly. It was also essential that I take off my glasses and, when I was done, kiss the bottom knuckles of my thumbs three times. It was a kind of obsessive-compulsive ritual, a distraction. At first I prayed to God to save my life. Then I started proposing more limited offers: Let me see A.J.'s high school graduation. How about college? Her wedding?

I latched onto weird, totemic things. Didi's mom had traveled to Beijing to play a concert and brought me a little Buddha. I would rub the top of its head for luck. (I was an equal opportunity religion adopter.) Didi bought me a stuffed tiger from a hospital gift shop. I carried it in my briefcase every day. Not that I believe in the power of it or anything, but I still have it.

In November, a few days after I was diagnosed, I went to a Korean deli near my office for lunch. I bought a sandwich, a soda, and a bag of pretzels, and when the woman at the cash register rang me up, the total came to $6.66. She didn't know I had cancer, of course, but she nevertheless thought it was spooky. She immediately punched another one-cent charge into the cash register to change the total to $6.67.

4.

IF YOU HAVEN'T had cancer before, you imagine, at first, that diagnosing it is like diagnosing any other disease: You take a test, and it comes up positive or negative, and you either have the thing or you don't. But cancer isn't strep throat. There are thousands of cancers with hundreds of overlapping markers and symptoms, many of them difficult to identify. Most people have never even heard of multiple myeloma (when I tell people what I have, they often think I say "melanoma," as in skin cancer), and it has numerous subtypes of its own. To determine exactly what kind of cancer you have, you often have to have a constellation of tests, no one of which is conclusive. The doctors gather puzzle pieces and put them together until a coherent picture emerges.

My initial diagnosis took three primary doctors, plus radiologists, imaging and lab technicians, and doctors consulted for second opinions; dozens of blood tests, biopsies, X-rays, MRIs, CT scans, and PET scans; and two and a half months. It also changed radically along the way. As advanced as modern medicine is, we are still light-years away from the *Star Trek* vision of instantaneous, noninvasive diagnosis by Tricorder. Although artificial intelligence promises to speed diagnoses and make them more accurate, it doesn't prevent the need for blood draws, biopsies, and scans.

Because the MRI report suggested that bone cancer was my diagnosis, Dr. Weiner referred me to Dr. Patrick Boland, a specialist in that condition at Memorial Sloan Kettering Cancer Center, one of the world's top cancer hospitals.

Before I got sick, I thought about medical insurance, if I thought about it at all, as a social or political issue, not a personal one. Because I was lucky enough to have a job, I had employer-based coverage. Because I was lucky enough to be well, I needed only routine doctors appointments and tests that I could comfortably afford. Generally speaking, I was happy to see providers in my network, whoever they were, and if I had to go out of network, the portion of the payment I was responsible for didn't amount to much.

Now I was in a different world. Where I received my care could be potentially a matter of life or death, and that care was going to be expensive. Going "out of network" could cost hundreds, thousands, or tens of thousands of dollars.

In what would turn out to be just the first of hundreds of infuriating insurance hassles I would experience over the next twenty-plus years, Sloan Kettering didn't take my insurance.

I was fortunate to have medical insurance at all. As of 2023, some 25 million Americans were uninsured, which can have devastating effects. Uninsured people are less likely to receive preventive services for chronic conditions such as cancer, cardiovascular disease, and diabetes. Because people who are uninsured are also less likely than those who are insured to receive follow-up screenings, the uninsured have an increased risk of being diagnosed at later stages of diseases and have higher mortality rates than those with insurance. More than 65 percent of bankruptcies are caused directly by medical expenses, making them the number one cause of bankruptcy.

Our national healthcare system is problematic enough if you're healthy and employed. If you're sick and out of work, it is a recipe for otherwise preventable illness, premature death, and financial ruin. Those of us who carry an insurance card in our wallets are lucky indeed. It is more than a thin strip of plastic; it is a ticket to a better life.

Despite the fact that Dr. Boland didn't take my insurance, Didi and I decided I would see him. It was critical that I get the correct diagnosis, and it was clear that Dr. Boland was a leading figure in his field. Because it was just a consultation, the cost difference between an in-network and out-of-network visit was minimal. An extra couple of hundred dollars seemed like a reasonable price to pay for a potentially lifesaving diagnosis.

To determine exactly what kind of tumor I had, Dr. Boland ordered something called a CT-guided bone biopsy. Sloan Kettering was clearly an excellent place to have it done. Some of the most skilled cancer experts in the world worked there, and Dr. Boland could order the test and get access to the results without third parties being involved. But because a CT-guided biopsy is considerably more expensive than a standard doctor's office visit and because Dr. Boland assured us that it was a relatively routine procedure, Didi and I decided I would have it done in network at Lenox Hill.

5.

TO PERFORM A CT-guided bone biopsy, a nurse sets you up with IV sedatives and numbs the area in question with a local anesthetic. Then the doctor inserts a needle through your skin until the tip is positioned against the surface of the bone. At that point, a technician slides you into and out of the CT scanner to see if the needle is in the correct spot. Because of the anesthetic, positioning the needle doesn't hurt much. But because the anesthetic doesn't numb the bone, removal of the bone tissue is painful. A special drill needle is used that has a hollow core to capture the bone specimen. You feel the needle pressing on the surface of bone; then you feel a pop when it breaks through the surface. The pop is accompanied by a stab of sharp pain. Next you feel a grinding sensation as the bone tissue is extracted. The technician re-moves the needle, places the specimen in a test tube, and sends it to the lab.

When I went to see Dr. Boland for the results of my test, I ran into him in the hallway; he was carrying the lab report. He hadn't read it yet, so he opened it on the spot. The rele-vant language read, "Suspect a plasma cell neoplasm."

As I had done with Dr. Weiner, I asked Dr. Boland to translate the medical-speak into lay terms. He explained that it appeared I had a form of bone marrow cancer, not bone cancer. It might be isolated to the lesion on my hip, in which case it would be classified as something called a solitary plas-macytoma, or it might be the first manifestation of some-thing called multiple myeloma, a disease of the plasma cells that can damage the bones, kidneys, and immune system.

Multiple myeloma is incurable, he said. Although it can typically be put into remission, in some cases numerous times, it will, almost without fail, recur. A solitary plasma-cytoma, on the other hand, can sometimes be treated and not return, he said. The catch, he explained, is that a solitary plasmacytoma almost always turns into multiple myeloma.

To avoid coming across upsetting or inaccurate informa-tion, I had been warned by a number of people not to go on the internet, to just "trust my doctors." But I am inquisitive by nature and a journalist by profession. Not knowing things makes me anxious, and knowing them gives me a feeling, however illusory, of control. That night, after Didi and A.J. went to sleep, I logged on to my computer.

Within minutes, I learned that solitary plasmacytomas are highly treatable when they occur in soft tissue but much less treatable, and more likely to develop into myeloma, when they occur in bone. I learned about the disease's dismal survival rates. And I stumbled across pictures of myeloma patients' X-rays in which their bones looked like Swiss cheese. I logged off.

6.

IN THE YEARS since, I have learned a great deal more about solitary plasmacytomas and multiple myeloma. At root, both conditions are diseases of plasma cells, a type of white blood cell that's a critical component of the human immune system. Like all other cells, plasma cells are produced in the bone marrow, the spongy tissue inside our bones. Our immune systems produce both short-lived and long-lived versions of plasma cells; their respective lifespans are what enable them to provide both immediate and prolonged protection from infections. Long-lived plasma cells remain mainly in bone marrow, whose specialized and protected environment enables them to survive for decades or longer. Short-lived plasma cells, which make up the majority of plasma cells, circulate in the blood and lymphatic systems.

Short-lived plasma cells are produced on demand, as a response to the presence of foreign invaders, most commonly infectious pathogens such as bacteria, viruses, parasites, or fungi. These invaders have specific molecules on their surfaces referred to as antigens. Think of an antigen as the keyhole in a cellular lock. When the body detects an invader, it produces short-term plasma cells. Each plasma cell can secrete thousands of copies of a specific protein, called an antibody, which fits like a key into the antigen, or cellular keyhole, of the invader.

Once the key is in the lock, the antibody marks the invading cell for destruction by other components of the immune system. The defensive response of plasma cells then subsides once the threat is overcome. That can be in a matter of days, in the case of an acute infection, or longer if the infection is persistent or more difficult to subdue.

At its root, cancer is a disease of abnormal cell growth. In healthy cells, fundamental genetic signals regulate cell division and cell death. In cancer cells, DNA mutations cause that mechanism to malfunction, triggering uncontrolled and destructive growth.

That fine line between healthy and unhealthy cell growth has profound implications. As Siddhartha Mukherjee wrote in his Pulitzer Prize–winning *The Emperor of All Maladies: A Biography of Cancer,* "That this seemingly simple mechanism—cell growth without barriers—can lie at the heart of this grotesque and multifaceted illness is a testament to the unfathomable power of cell growth. . . . Cancer cells grow faster, adapt better. They are more perfect versions of ourselves."

A neoplasm is an abnormal proliferation of cells. While neoplasms are sometimes benign, most are either cancerous or precancerous. Neoplasms that affect white blood cells include myeloma, as well as leukemia and lymphoma; other neoplasms impact red blood cells or platelets. In all blood or bone marrow cancers (and multiple myeloma can be described as either), the burgeoning numbers of abnormal blood cells crowd out the normal cells in the marrow. As a result, there are not enough healthy cells to carry out their normal functions.

Myeloma cells attack the body on several fronts. The cancerous plasma cells produce large amounts of an abnormal antibody, variously referred to as M protein, myeloma protein, or M spike, which does not help fight infection but rather builds up in bone marrow and forms tumors in bones, like the one in my hip. The destruction of bone tissue, in turn, releases calcium into circulation, which can result in kidney stress. At the same time, M proteins can cause the blood to thicken and concentrate in urine, both of which can cause renal problems. Myeloma cells can also cause a reduction in overall blood cell counts, which can lead to anemia, and in normal antibodies, which can lead to compromised immunity and an increased risk of infections. The criteria for diagnosing myeloma are sometimes described using the acronym CRAB: Calcium elevation, Renal issues, Anemia, Bone problems.

A variety of tests are used to determine if a patient has myeloma: blood chemistry measures, including M protein, blood calcium, and antibody levels; kidney function and anemia tests; imaging exams, including X-rays, CT, MRI, and/or PET scans; and bone and bone marrow biopsies. Not all signs and symptoms of the disease need to be present to constitute a myeloma diagnosis, and the thresholds of the various diagnostic measures also matter.

The same is true for staging multiple myeloma. Doctors use an array of measures to determine the stage of the disease, with the stages ranging from Stage 1 to Stage 3. In myeloma, the staging system is used only for newly diagnosed patients, with Stage 1 representing the lowest risk type of the disease and Stage 3 the highest.

Once a diagnosis of multiple myeloma is made, treatment typically starts right away. What treatments are used depends on what stage the disease is at, a patient's age and health, and what treatments they have had previously, among other factors. Having not yet received a definitive diagnosis, I was just at the start of that journey.

7.

MY OLDEST SISTER, Jennifer, is a social worker who works at a school for children with social, emotional, and behavioral challenges. She lives in Katonah, New York, about an hour north of New York City, and has two grown sons. She is a savant of a listener. My sister Tina is a retired math teacher and tutor who specialized in helping young girls develop self-esteem. She and her husband, Paul, live in Boston. They have three adult children, two girls on either end of the age spectrum and a boy in the middle. Tina is empathic; she hurts for you when something hurts. My brother, Andy, and his wife, Kim, live in Newton, Massachusetts, a suburb of Boston. Andy is a teacher's aide who spent seventeen years working at the elementary school his daughter and son attended before retiring. He is a legitimate candidate for world's most optimistic human. My mother, Betsy, is famously sunny, and my father, Gene, was preternaturally calm.

When I called each of them to tell them I had cancer, they all reacted accordingly. My mother predicted a happy ending: "We're going to beat this!" My father was even-keeled and reassuring: "We hear you, son. We understand." Jen said she was sorry, Tina was audibly pained, and Andy was brimming with positivity. Everyone offered to help in any way they could.

Who knows how they really felt or what they said to one another or their families or friends after we hung up, but that was the show they put on for me, and I was grateful for it. One of the hardest things about getting sick is that you feel as though you're upsetting the people who love you and care about you. It may not be your fault, but you still feel responsible—and guilty.

Not everyone I told about my illness responded so helpfully. Several people felt compelled to tell me stories about friends who had had a solitary plasmacytoma or multiple myeloma and died. One friend told me she understood what I was going through, then proceeded to tell me about a forty-eight-hour skin cancer scare that had turned out to be nothing. A taxi driver noticed that I was limping, asked what was wrong, then browbeat me for my foolish reliance on Western medicine. Several people said they "knew" I would be okay.

The truth is, a simple expression of warmth or sympathy went a long way. One coworker said, "You poor guy. I'm sorry." That was about right. My best friend from childhood sent me a letter. Near the end he wrote, "You are my oldest friend." I don't know why that had so much power, but for the first time since I'd found out I had cancer, I burst into tears.

8.

NOW THAT I knew I had bone marrow cancer, I needed a new doctor. I went to see Dr. Steven Gruenstein, a hematologist and oncologist at Mount Sinai, another top cancer hospital. New York may be loud, crowded, expensive, and many other unwelcome things, but there is no better place to live if you need an oncologist.

Dr. Gruenstein is a big, lovable bear of a man, the son every stereotypical Jewish mother dreams about. He is a cancer survivor himself, kidney cancer.

His first job, he said, was to confirm that I had a solitary plasmacytoma and not multiple myeloma. To do that, he would need to perform a variety of blood tests, urine tests, imaging tests, and a bone marrow biopsy.

A bone marrow biopsy is similar to a bone biopsy, only the needle is inserted not just into the bone but through the bone and into the marrow, and a sample of the marrow, not the bone, is extracted. In multiple myeloma, a bone marrow biopsy provides information about how prevalent and aggressive the disease is. It can also detect genetic abnormalities that can help determine treatment choices and predict the disease's course.

Dr. Gruenstein performed the procedure on the spot, in one of his examining rooms, and sent me home with a cane. The tumor was threatening to breach the exterior wall of my pelvic bone, he said, and he was concerned that I might fracture it.

Two days later, he called me with my test results. The biopsy was inconclusive—the sample was "hypocellular"; it didn't contain enough cells to get a valid reading. I'd have to do it again.

I was angry at first; I thought that Dr. Gruenstein had mishandled the procedure. But it turned out that that result isn't uncommon. Still, I had to endure another biopsy. That one also came back hypocellular, as did a third one.

I was beginning to feel like a pin cushion or maybe, more accurately, like a stuck pig. Between biopsies, blood draws, IV infusions, and other procedures that involve being poked with needles, it was a feeling I would go on to have thousands of times. Although I don't especially mind needles, I can't say I enjoy them, either. In any case, fewer is better than more.

Bone marrow biopsies are generally performed in the top, backward-facing portion of the pelvic bone. That area is large enough and strong enough to withstand the pressure required to insert the biopsy needle without fracturing; it contains a substantial reserve of marrow, and if the needle slips or penetrates farther than intended, it won't hit a vital organ. You lie on your stomach to have the procedure done.

Because my pelvic bone didn't seem to be cooperating (we had tried both sides), Dr. Gruenstein suggested a variation of the procedure called a sternum biopsy. Like your hip bone, your sternum is strong and has plenty of marrow. Unlike your hip bone, it is located in the vicinity of your heart and lungs. Because of the added risk involved and because Dr. Gruenstein hadn't performed many sternum biopsies, he asked one of his colleagues to perform the procedure.

Several days later, Dr. Gruenstein called to say that the sternum biopsy had worked; the sample was viable. More important, it contained no detectable myeloma cells. So far, I still had a solitary plasmacytoma and not multiple myeloma.

Next, Dr. Gruenstein ordered a full-body PET scan. X-rays, MRIs, and CT scans can "see" anomalous spots in bones and soft tissue, but they can't detect metabolic activity. A PET scan can. In the procedure, a radioactive tracer is injected into your bloodstream. After waiting forty-five minutes for the solution to circulate throughout your body, you lie down on a machine similar to a CT scanner and are slowly passed through it (a full-body PET scan typically takes twenty to thirty minutes to complete). Because cancer cells "take up" the radioactive tracer faster than other cells do, malignancies light up.

Never mind that a PET scan is considered one of the most valuable tests for multiple myeloma and that detecting the disease early might add years to my life. Oxford, my insurance company, refused to pay for it. In its twisted logic, I had no evidence of multiple myeloma from the tests I'd done so far, so I didn't have it. No further testing was needed. It was the first of what would turn out to be many insurance battles I would fight over so-called pre-authorization.

Pre-authorization, or "pre-auth," is an attempt on the part

of insurance companies to limit unnecessary tests, medications, treatments, and procedures. Before insurers will agree to pay for certain items, especially high-cost or high-risk ones, the companies' in-house medical experts review them to determine whether the company considers them necessary. If so, the procedure is approved. If not, not.

In theory, the system exists to protect patients from undergoing unnecessary tests, treatments, or procedures and to keep healthcare costs in check. In practice, it can be used as a way for insurance companies to boost their profits. Pre-authorization also creates red tape and can slow down, if not block, patients' access to healthcare.

Beginning with that PET scan decision and continuing to this day, I have had to appeal scores of pre-authorization denials. As anyone who has gone through the process knows, it can be Kafkaesque. Essentially, your doctor needs to convince the insurance company that the test or treatment in question is, in fact, necessary. That involves the doctor's office sending a letter to the insurance company making that case, along with the appropriate medical records.

The process can take days or weeks under the best of circumstances, and as often as not something goes wrong. The doctor forgets to ask the pre-auth coordinator to make the request. The pre-auth coordinator is slow to pursue the matter or forgets about it altogether. The doctor's argument isn't convincing. The insurance company is slow to respond. All of those things and more have happened to me.

Ultimately the burden falls on the patient to resolve any difficulties. The time it takes and the stress it brings can be considerable. You often have to call the doctor's office and the insurance company repeatedly. You spend countless hours on hold. You are directed to the wrong person or department. Unfortunately, the person you reach isn't sure why the procedure was denied. Yes, that does make it impossible for your doctor to appeal the case . . . Yes, they understand you're frustrated and angry . . . No, there's nothing else they can do at this time. Blah, blah, blah.

I have spent hundreds of hours fighting pre-authorization battles and have tried every tactic I can think of—calm reasoning, obsequious kindness, screaming—to resolve them.

What I have discovered is that the person on the other end of the line has to care. Sometimes they do, sometimes they don't. It turns out that the secret to navigating the pre-authorization maze, and the American health insurance system in general, is to cross your fingers and hope.

People sometimes ask me, "Doesn't cancer ever make you angry?" Ask a pre-auth representative at Oxford.

Not that Oxford is the only offender. As I changed jobs or my employers changed insurers, I would go on to have equally frustrating experiences with a whole alphabet soup of insurance companies: Aetna, Anthem, Blue Cross, Cigna, Oxford, and UnitedHealthcare. I can't say I recommend any of them. Medical insurers are like airlines: The worst one is the one you're using.

In keeping with the pre-authorization protocols, Dr. Gruenstein wrote a letter of appeal regarding my PET scan, and after several weeks of waiting, the procedure was finally approved.

I had the exam done after work one night. Afterward, when I had changed from my gown back into my street clothes and was on my way out, I tried to peek at the scan on the monitor in the technician's office. That was useless. I had no idea what the jumble of shapes and colors meant—to my eye, it was essentially a two-year-old's finger painting—or even if it was my scan.

I asked the technician if he could share anything about what he saw, but he told me that wasn't allowed; my doctor would call me with the results within forty-eight hours. I tried to read his expression, but that was also futile. He had seen the likes of me before. He was poker-faced. As I put on my coat and made my way to the door, I asked the technician if I was glowing from the radioactive tracer. I meant it as a bit of gallows humor, but he answered by essentially saying, "Actually, sort of."

He told me that the isotope has a half-life of about six hours. It wasn't strictly necessary, he said, but I might want to avoid sleeping next to my wife tonight, especially if she was pregnant. I told him that my wife wasn't pregnant, but we had a seven-month-old daughter. "Oh," he said. "You should definitely stay away from her."

By some estimates, overt medical errors—misdiagnoses, dangerous drug interactions, botched surgeries—play a part in almost 100,000 deaths in the United States each year, with some reports putting that number at more than 400,000.

But doctors and other medical professionals also commit errors of omission. What would have happened if I hadn't made that joke to the PET scan technician? Why wasn't I warned of the potential risks to Didi and A.J.? What similar hazards have I, or you, not been informed of? There's no way to know.

That night, I went to a diner, had a cheeseburger deluxe, and stayed there and read until 2:00 A.M. Because I was afraid of irradiating someone next to me, I sat alone. I felt like a character in an Edward Hopper painting.

9.

THE LAST HURDLE in the diagnostic gauntlet I was running was something called a twenty-four-hour urine test. Used to determine the level of M protein in your urine and whether your kidneys are functioning properly, the test is exactly what it sounds like. For a full day, every time you have to urinate, you do so into a large plastic jug that looks vaguely like a laundry detergent bottle. To produce the most accurate results, the container needs to be refrigerated. That day, every time Didi or I went for a glass of orange juice, the leftover lo mein noodles, or a bottle of milk for A.J., there was cancer, sitting in our fridge.

10.

ON THURSDAY, DECEMBER 11, a month and a week after I was told I had cancer, I met with Dr. Gruenstein in his office. Based on all the tests he had done, he said he believed I had a solitary plasmacytoma, not multiple myeloma, and that he could put it into remission.

Remission for a day? A month? A year? Forever? He couldn't say.

I asked what the odds were of its eventually developing into multiple myeloma. Again, there was no firm answer.

The good news, he said, was that I wouldn't need surgery or chemotherapy. He also mentioned that multiple myeloma had recently become an area of intense research and that there were a number of promising new drugs in the pipeline. For now, he said, radiation was the indicated treatment.

What were the chances it would work? He couldn't tell me that, either. "It's not a pipe dream," he said, nor was there a guarantee. We would have to wait and see.

11.

I MENTIONED THAT Didi wasn't outwardly emotional about any of it, and that I liked that. That was true. Her strength gave me strength. Her calm kept me calm. Yet at the same time, I had begun to wonder: If she never gets upset, does she care?

After a while, I started to resent the fact that she hadn't had a meltdown. What kind of person doesn't dissolve into a puddle of tears or break down when their spouse is diagnosed with cancer? Is she heartless? Does she not love me? These are the kinds of questions that can start to eat at a relationship touched by cancer.

One day my anger boiled over. Why wasn't Didi more upset? What was *wrong* with her? Didi kept her cool. She explained that she cared but couldn't afford to let her emotions go. She had too much on her own plate to allow herself to do that, at least for the time being.

In the years since we had moved to New York, Didi had worked at a number of women's magazines: *Ladies' Home Journal, Good Housekeeping, Redbook.* Now she was working at *Marie Claire,* trying to balance the demands of her career with new motherhood. A.J. was still just seven months old, and Didi was still nursing. (We had a nanny who took care of A.J. during the day.) Just as I was facing frightening thoughts from being sick, Didi was confronted with scary questions resulting from being married to someone who was sick: What would she do if I died? Would she be able to support herself and A.J.? Would she have to sell our apartment and move? She had already lost her father prematurely. Would she have to face a second, similar loss?

After A.J. was born, Didi's primary domestic focus had already shifted from me to the baby. Now, with the idea that she might become a single parent hovering in the air, her maternal instincts kicked in even harder. Her top priorities were to keep herself healthy and functioning and to care for and protect A.J.

I understood all of that. If anything, I didn't want to drag Didi and A.J. down into my illness. I already felt guilty enough about how my diagnosis might affect them. If Didi needed to keep her feelings in check for the time being for the sake of herself and our daughter, that was fine with me. That was how the rational side of me felt, anyway. The emotional side wanted the meltdown.

12.

NEW YORK MAGAZINE used to host something called the *New York* Awards in mid-December. That year, the event was held at a luncheon at the Four Seasons restaurant. Hillary Clinton, Caroline Kennedy, and Kevin Kline were among the honorees. Meryl Streep, a friend of Kline's, was asked to present his award. The woman who coordinated the event knew I was sick and let me choose who I wanted to sit next to. As a fan of her work, I chose Streep.

The world's greatest actress and I were introduced at the cocktail reception, and when she saw my cane, she asked me what the problem was.

"I've got a bum hip," I said, hoping she'd leave it at that.

"What happened?" she asked.

"It's a long story," I said.

I kept trying to change the subject, but she wouldn't stop asking about my hip. Finally, I ran out of bullshit answers and blurted out, "Actually, I have bone marrow cancer. There's a tumor on my hip."

I can tell you that Meryl Streep is either the most sincere person in the world or an even better actor than we all know. What she did was reach over, put her hand on my forearm, look into my eyes, and somehow convey more genuine human concern than anyone else I've ever known.

Later, as we were saying our goodbyes, she wished me the best. I responded with some throwaway remark such as "What are you going to do?" And she looked at me again with that look, the close-up-at-the-end-of-the-third-reel look, and said, "That's what life is. Shit happens, and you deal with it." Buddhism by Streep.

13.

DIDI AND I have tried, but we can't remember what she, A.J., and I did for the holidays that year. It's a blank. What we do recall is spending most of December and January dealing with our new reality.

The previous winter, in anticipation of A.J. being born, Didi and I had taken out life insurance policies. It was a good thing we did because my diagnosis would have disqualified me or made the coverage prohibitively expensive. (This was before the Affordable Care Act prohibited insurers from denying coverage to people with preexisting conditions.) Through a combination of new-parent-to-be planning and pure luck, we had that base covered. What we hadn't gotten around to was drawing up wills. We were young and healthy; even with A.J. on the way, it hadn't seemed like a priority. Now it was.

We found a lawyer through a friend and met him in his midtown Manhattan office at lunch one day. He was a kindly older gentleman with a ring of white hair circling his otherwise bald head. We told him why we were there; then the three of us worked our way through the particulars: executors, beneficiaries, Do Not Resuscitate orders, healthcare proxies. He seemed to be moved by our story. Despite the fact that he was a virtual stranger, there was something comforting about that. Like a good doctor, a good estate attorney has a reassuring bedside manner.

14.

NEXT, DIDI AND I had fertility questions to contend with. We had always agreed that we wanted at least one child and no more than two. We were well aware of how lucky we were to have A.J., but now, if we wanted to consider having a second child, I'd have to bank my sperm. Being radiated in my hip wasn't certain to leave me infertile, but it might.

Didi and I had one of those conversations a couple never thinks they'll have. The gist of it was: If I die, would you rather have just A.J. or A.J. and someone else? We punted and decided that for a couple of hundred dollars in handling and storage fees and a few minutes spent watching a bad porn VHS tape, I might as well go ahead and freeze my sperm. We could decide another time whether to use them.

On December 16, 2003, a clear and sunny Tuesday, I found myself leaving work at lunchtime and walking from my office on Madison and Forty-ninth to a fertility clinic on Park Avenue South. I called my sister Jen, with whom I share a dark sense of humor, and said, "Okay, this is what it's come down to. I'm thirty-eight years old. I have cancer. I have to have radiation therapy, which may or may not make me better, and I'm about to go jerk off on Park Avenue."

15.

I ALSO NEEDED to do something called a stem cell harvest. Should my disease develop into multiple myeloma, I might need a bone marrow transplant.

Patients in need of such a transplant can get marrow from a donor, but finding a match can be difficult. To help address that problem, doctors have developed an alternative: Technicians harvest your stem cells and freeze them so you can, in effect, give yourself a transplant—a stem cell transplant. (Although the terms "bone marrow transplant" and "stem cell transplant" are sometimes used interchangeably, the latter is technically a subset of the former. The main difference is that the stem cells used in a bone marrow transplant come from the bone marrow, while stem cells used for a stem cell transplant can also come from peripheral blood or umbilical cord blood.)

Stem cells are cells that produce other blood cells, including red cells, white cells, and platelets. In some cancers, the chemotherapy or other treatment typically administered before a bone marrow or stem cell transplant permanently destroys the malignancy, and the transplant results in a cure, once the transplanted cells produce healthy new cells. Multiple myeloma is not one of those cancers. With myeloma, the transplanted cells give you a restart, but that's all. They're not curative; the cancer eventually returns. The best a transplant can do for myeloma patients is buy them time.

On December 19, 2003, I saw Dr. Luis Isola, a marrow transplant specialist at Mount Sinai. In Dr. Isola's waiting room, there was a loud middle-aged woman who was talking to the woman next to her. She blurted out, in full voice, "Yes, but they caught it too late, and it ate through her spine." From that point on, I started wearing headphones to my appointments.

To prepare for a stem cell harvest, you inject yourself with a drug called Neupogen, which boosts your stem cell count, for three days prior. A nurse gives you a little kit and teaches you how to give yourself the shots. Like a twenty-four-hour urine sample, Neupogen has to be stored in the refrigerator. Because it comes in small white boxes, at least I could keep it out of sight, in the crisper.

On the morning of January 26, 2004, Didi and I took a cab to Mount Sinai for the stem cell harvest. In the procedure, known as apheresis, technicians use a Frankensteinian-looking machine to take the blood out of one arm, remove the stem cells, then pump the remaining blood back into your other arm. The process can cause a drop in your calcium level, I'd been told, which can make you tingle. What I experienced was more like a fire ant attack. The technicians started pumping me full of yogurt, but it didn't really help. I lost the feeling in my feet and couldn't walk. Eight hours and a half-dozen cups of Dannon lemon flavor later, Didi helped me get into a cab.

By now I was limping badly and using the cane all the time. On my way to and from work, I somehow expected that people on the subway would offer me a seat, but almost no one cut me any slack. The city was going to make me fight for my position in it, just as it always had. Perhaps this is a pathology unique to being a New Yorker, but I kind of liked that.

16.

A SHORT TIME later, New York magazine hired a new editor in chief, Adam Moss, who had previously been the editor of The New York Times Magazine. Owing to a merry-go-round of ownership changes over the years, New York had strayed from its original mission and lost some of its cachet. When yet another new owner took control of the publication, he hired Adam to revitalize it.

Because I would have to be out of the office for several hours a day to get my radiation treatments, I had no choice but to tell Adam what was going on. But I also told him I didn't expect my treatments to be terribly debilitating and I asked him to treat me the same way he would treat anyone else. If I needed any sort of accommodation, I told him, I would ask. Whatever else I was, I didn't want to be a sympathy case.

Adam said he was sorry, that he was familiar with multiple myeloma, and that he would honor my request. At the same time, Adam is not the type to compromise his standards. He is not unreasonable—in fact, he has a gentle personal manner—but he is committed to producing the best work he can and expects everyone who works for him to do the same. What that meant for those of us at *New York* was that we were essentially auditioning for our jobs.

17.

BEFORE I STARTED my radiation treatments, I decided to get a second opinion. In my internet research, I had come across a doctor named Sundar Jagannath, a world-renowned multiple myeloma expert who was at the time the head of the multiple myeloma program at St. Vincent's Hospital in New York, just a few blocks from my apartment.

That February, I saw Dr. Jagannath. A reed-thin Indian American man with a push-broom mustache, Dr. Jagannath has the air of a friendly supercomputer. His caring and expertise are immediately evident. When he agreed that I had a solitary plasmacytoma and the best treatment would be localized radiation, I felt confident that I was on the right path. It was time to get started.

18.

RADIATION THERAPY DATES back more than 130 years to the discovery of the X-ray in 1896 by the German physicist Wilhelm Conrad Röntgen. Within several years of the development of that technology, radiation was being used to treat breast, skin, and stomach cancers, and in 1901, Röntgen was awarded the first Nobel Prize in Physics.

Soon thereafter, doctors in France found that administering daily doses of radiation over several weeks was particularly effective, but dosing was still not well understood and targeting techniques were primitive. At around the same time, doctors discovered that radiation could *cause* cancer, in addition to curing it, underscoring the need for more nuanced treatment methods.

Radiation techniques improved steadily throughout the ensuing years, and quantum leaps in imaging technology and computing in the latter part of the twentieth century made it possible to administer radiation more safely and effectively.

A technique called conformal radiation therapy, for example, allows doctors to pinpoint the location of a tumor in three dimensions and deliver a radiation dose from multiple directions in the exact shape of the tumor. And a technology called conformal proton beam radiation therapy uses proton beams instead of X-rays to target malignancies. Because protons (parts of atoms) cause less damage than X-rays to the tissues they pass through, the technology allows doctors to deliver a larger dose of radiation to the area in question while minimizing damage to other parts of the body.

To plan my radiation treatment, I met with Dr. Jack Dalton, a radiation oncologist at Mount Sinai, and he laid out my protocol. (The subspecialties involved in cancer care can be confusing in their own right. Radiation oncologists specialize in that treatment per se. They are neither radiologists, who specialize in medical imaging, nor medical oncologists, who are what laypeople generally call oncologists.) Dr. Dalton said I would need to be radiated five days a week for five weeks, twenty-five sessions in all. He said that I might be tired but I shouldn't be nauseous and that I should be able to go to work every day. He said I might have skin burns on the area being radiated and perhaps diarrhea or other lower GI issues, but that was about it in terms of short-term side effects. I wouldn't lose my hair. He also told me that he would build a sort of jury-rigged athletic cup–type device to try to preserve my fertility, but he couldn't guarantee that it would work. Stray radiation bounces around inside the body somewhat.

As a next step, I had to get "mapped." Before administering radiation therapy, technicians use a system of CT scans, X-rays, and lasers to precisely identify the area they're targeting in three dimensions. They then tattoo you with little blue dots to mark the area that's being radiated so they don't have to relocate it on each day of your treatment.

As with the marrow biopsies, there was a glitch in the imaging portion of my mapping session, and it had to be repeated. Fortunately, the tattoos aren't done until the imaging portion of the process is successfully completed. The second session worked, and I got my tats.

19.

I HAD MY first radiation session on February 9, 2004, fully three months after Dr. Weiner had told me I had cancer. The treatments themselves were surprisingly unremarkable. You lie down on the table of what looks like a giant X-ray machine. A technician uses lasers and your tattoos to line up the radiation beam, then swings a large device over you that looks like a TV satellite dish that delivers the radiation into you for roughly thirty seconds. You don't feel anything. It's so painless, in fact, that I wondered from time to time if I weren't an unknowing participant in some kind of placebo experiment.

The Mount Sinai radiation oncology unit is in the basement, literally underground. Some of the sickest people I've seen anywhere, I saw there. It's like a ghost world; you realize that there's a whole shadow population of sick people who are shunted around out of view. Maybe that's healthy; maybe it would be too much to have to stare at the ugly side of life every day. Or maybe we're callous and afraid.

As Dr. Dalton had predicted, I was a little tired and I experienced skin burns and diarrhea. But for the most part, I felt surprisingly well and worked every day during my treatment. It's almost a cancer cliché: "He didn't miss a day of work. How brave." Believe me, it has nothing to do with bravery, at least not in my case. In my case, it had to do with terror: I could sit home and contemplate the dimming of the light or go to work and edit stories about misbehaving politicians or new sushi restaurants. For me, the choice was obvious.

About a month after my last radiation treatment, I met with Dr. Gruenstein for my first postradiation checkup. He told me he wanted to do an M protein test but warned me that it was too early to expect the number to have returned to normal. For now, he wanted to be sure the number hadn't gone up (a possibility I somehow hadn't considered). I had the blood drawn that day and watched the technician carry off the vial. I would get the results in a week to ten days. "Make that a good one," I said.

20.

I WAS BORN on Saturday, April 17, 1965. On Friday, April 16, 2004, Dr. Gruenstein called to say that my M spike had returned to normal. I was in remission. Some cancer survivors call this your second birthday, but that term has always seemed a little goofy to me.

Here's the thing about cancer, or my cancer anyway: You know there is no cure, and you know you're not even considered de facto "cured" until you've been cancer free for five years. But when your oncologist calls and tells you that your radiation therapy has worked and that there is "no current evidence of disease" and that this is "the best possible outcome" from the radiation, well, what you do is you start thanking him like a blubbering fool and telling him you owe him your life but that you really need to get off the phone and call your wife and that you'll call him back tomorrow to discuss next steps, and then you hang up and shout "*Yes!*" right there at your desk, and then you call your wife and tell her the news and she says, "Holy shit! I knew it!" and you tell her that you could feel her confidence all along, and you thank her for being wise enough not to express that belief until now, and you can practically feel her exhale on the other end of the line, a big, giant cosmic exhale, and she's the one who first points out that this news has come on the day before your birthday, and she says we'll have to double celebrate tonight and the next night since we were planning on going out for your birthday anyway, and then you hang up and run around your office telling your boss and your boss's assistant and whoever else is in your lunatic path that, for the time being anyway, you are going to live and not die, and then you leave work immediately and go to meet your wife for your cancer-free celebration dinner.

Didi and I may not be especially religious, but we are Jews, and so we feel guilty. We go to expensive restaurants only on special occasions or for business lunches, and even then, we can have a hard time indulging. You would think that night would have been an exception, but the truth is, it wasn't. Our initial euphoria gave way to a set of more complicated emotions. The good news somehow also brought to the surface all the sadness and difficulty of the past year. Having only just set down a burden, we were exhausted. We had forgotten, in a sense, how to be happy.

My unconscious, however, was apparently less conflicted. The next morning, my thirty-ninth birthday, a song popped into my head that I didn't even know I knew the lyrics to. I was standing in the shower, and there it was: "I can see clearly now, the rain has gone. . . . It's gonna be a bright . . . bright . . . sunshiny day." I wouldn't blame anyone who doubts that it happened that way. Only it did.

But living with an incurable disease is like sleeping next to a hibernating bear. For the moment, I felt safe, but I knew it was only a matter of time before the bear woke up. And when it did, it would be hungry.

PART THREE

Limbo

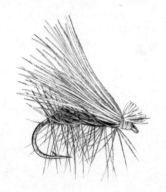

1 .

MOST CANCER STORIES take one of two forms: He or she fought valiantly and died or he or she fought valiantly and survived. The narrative of those of us who live with active cancers for unprecedented stretches traces its own arc. He or she fought valiantly, is still fighting, and will be fighting for as long as he or she lives. For some people who are diagnosed with cancer, the disease is a part of their life. For those of us destined to live with cancer as a permanent condition, it *is* our life.

So what do you do when you're told that you will be sick forever? That no one can say for sure how your illness will play out or how long you will survive? That there is no going back to your previous life, no matter how hard you pray or how earnestly you wish for that? How do you navigate that shocking new reality? How do you live with uncertainty when uncertainty isn't just something we all deal with some of the time but something you deal with all of the time?

Because cancer is a nuclear bomb, not a conventional weapon, the fallout is widespread. In my case, step one was to deal with the physical aftereffects.

Due to the damage to my pelvic bone, it was a year before Dr. Weiner, who was still overseeing my orthopedic care, cleared me to do even light exercise. During that period, I gained twenty pounds, and at an annual checkup with my general practitioner, I was told that my cholesterol level was high enough to warrant a Lipitor prescription. I pleaded for a reprieve on the premise that I could diet and exercise my way out of it, and my request was granted. I quickly lost sixteen pounds, four short of my precancer weight. I called it the Fear of Death Diet.

Because my radiation was localized, I didn't lose my hair, as Dr. Dalton had predicted. (Technically, I lost the hair in the area surrounding my hip but not the hair on my head.) And because the treatment effectively healed the hip lesion, I no longer needed a cane. (The pain in my hip lingered for a time but eventually subsided.) But because radiation therapy weakens your bones even as it heals them, I was told I could no longer run, play basketball, or ski, three things I loved to do. I was also told that I should avoid any activity, such as riding a bike or ice skating, where I might have a hard fall. If I broke my hip, which I was more prone than the average person to do, I could be facing a major disability.

The radiation also damaged the muscles around my hip. Despite the advances doctors have made in targeting and dosing radiation, the treatments still, in a sense, "cook" your muscles, leaving them less supple and flexible and more prone to stiffness, cramping, and pain. You could liken it to microwaving a steak. Once it's been zapped, it's never as tender.

As a form of preventive care, Dr. Gruenstein put me on a drug called Zometa (generic name zoledronic acid) that can help strengthen your bones and slow the damage myeloma does to them. But when reports surfaced that Zometa can cause something called osteonecrosis of the jaw, or ONJ, a type of bone death that can leave patients disabled or grossly disfigured, Dr. Gruenstein took me off the drug. (That a drug meant to strengthen my bones could cause my jawbone to disintegrate is not the kind of irony I appreciate.) The delicate balancing act of weighing how effective a cancer treatment is against its potentially serious side effects is one my doctors and I would have to perform again and again.

In compensating for the injury to my left hip, I developed arthritis in my right one. For a time, I took Vioxx, but that drug was taken off the market when it was found to pose a serious risk of stroke and heart attack.

People have asked me why I don't have my hip replaced. That procedure fixes the area where the top of the femur meets the pelvic bone. That's not where my tumor was; it was *in* my pelvic bone. As it doesn't replace the pelvic bone, a hip replacement would be pointless.

In the months following my remission, I got my teeth whitened, had my first-ever facial, and had two moles removed for strictly cosmetic reasons. Virtually no bodily imperfection, no matter how small, escaped my notice. I think I wanted to feel whole again.

2.

THAT WAS THE physical fallout from my diagnosis. Then there were the emotional aftereffects. Luckily, I had Dr. Gol to help with those.

I had first started seeing Dr. Gol to treat anxiety attacks I had been suffering from since I was a teenager. Improbably enough, I found her name in the yellow pages and called her because her office was three blocks from my apartment. I can't say that's the most advisable way to find a therapist, but for me it worked.

Dr. Gol has piercing blue eyes and close-cropped gray hair. She has the manner of a high mountain lake: deep and tranquil. She is wise. Her presence is calming. During the years she and I had been working together, we had engaged mostly in the slow, painstaking work of psychodynamic therapy—exploring my childhood and other past experiences and unpacking how they had influenced me. Because the benefits of that kind of therapy can be indirect and slow to reveal themselves, I would sometimes get frustrated and complain about the glacial speed at which we were progressing. But then I would realize that my anxiety was abating and therapy was making me feel happier and more stable, and I would drop my objections. Once or twice I quit my treatment, but I went back.

After my diagnosis, Dr. Gol and I continued to work on my long-term issues, but she would also sometimes suggest short-term techniques meant specifically to help me cope with the anxiety cancer brought. In one session shortly after I finished radiation, I told her I felt a pain in my thigh and couldn't stop worrying that my disease had come back.

"Stop," she said.

"What do you mean?"

"Stop the thought."

I thought she was joking, but she was teaching me a deceptively simple mental trick called thought stopping. When your mind starts to spin out of control, you tell yourself to stop. Then you replace the problematic thought with one you've prepared ahead of time, a simple phrase or song lyric, say. The method is by no means foolproof, but it can help. Just recognizing that I was spiraling helped me break the obsession circuit.

On another occasion, I was experiencing pain in my mid-back. After the third or fourth session in which I mentioned that I was worried about it and hemmed and hawed about whether I should get it checked out, Dr. Gol suggested that I see Dr. Gruenstein as soon as I could. The faster you get an answer, the faster you can close the rumination loop, she said. I saw Dr. Gruenstein and had an MRI that turned out to be negative. The next day, the pain went away.

In another session, I turned a small problem (one of my vaccinations was out-of-date) into a big one ("I'm going to

die from pneumonia because I'm weak from cancer and radiation!"). Dr. Gol helped teach me to avoid that kind of
"catastrophizing." She introduced me to the idea that
whether you feel good or bad at any given moment isn't a
black-or-white proposition. You can feel anxious without
coming unhinged. You can feel sad without becoming depressed. You can feel sick without thinking you're going to
die. She taught me a helpful mantra: "You don't have to feel
perfect to feel good."

Whenever I shared one cancer-related fear or another, Dr.
Gol would ask what exactly I was afraid of. What, specifically, was I worried might happen? Just naming your fears
and talking about them, she showed me, can diminish their
power. It can also help you see that your fears are often unwarranted. In another session in which I was worrying that
my disease would come back, she asked me what I was scared
of. When I said "Dying," she reminded me that my doctors
had told me there were many more treatments I could still
undergo and new ones in the works that could very well keep
me alive for a long time. That reality check helped arrest my
tailspin.

Immediately after I was told I was cancer free, I began
undergoing a surveillance regimen worthy of the Stasi—
MRIs, CT scans, PET scans, bone marrow biopsies, and an
array of complex blood work every three to six months—
that I still go through today. After every protein test, I still
have to wait for up to a week for the results. After every PET
scan, I still haunt some diner or coffee shop for a few hours
and read.

Dr. Gol suggested some ways to help me get through those
testing periods. She suggested that I avoid scheduling scans
on Fridays so I didn't have to wait two extra days to get the

results, and that when it was time for my tests, I book them as soon as I could to get them over with. As simple as those ideas sound, they helped.

When I used the word *chemo* once, Dr. Gol suggested I might want to abandon that term in favor of the more formal "chemotherapy." She thought "chemo" was too familiar. Cancer is like an unwelcome houseguest, she said. You don't want to be too friendly to it, or it might come back.

Occasionally, our discussions about my illness led me to a deeper, more far-reaching insight. Dr. Gol helped me see that illness can be a helpful corrective for narcissism. If you're so important, why is the universe so indifferent to you? If you're so powerful, why can't you fix this?

Shortly after I was diagnosed, Dr. Gol suggested I seek out a support group. She referred me to an organization called Gilda's Club, a community center founded in downtown Manhattan by friends and family members of the late *Saturday Night Live* star Gilda Radner after Radner was diagnosed with ovarian cancer.

Gilda's Club, which has since changed its name to Red Door Community, organizes its support groups by cancer type, and I signed up for a "blood cancers" session. The meeting I attended was led by a lymphoma survivor named Jonathan, who began the evening by sharing his story.

It turned out that group therapy wasn't for me. By nature, I'm not a joiner, and frankly some of the things I heard that night scared me. Nevertheless, meeting Jonathan and hearing his story had a powerful effect. It's not as though I didn't know that surviving cancer was possible, but Jonathan was the first cancer survivor I had met since my diagnosis. And the fact that we shared a first name was somehow meaningful to me. The other Jonathan had undergone radiation therapy, chemotherapy, and a bone marrow transplant, far more treatment than I had been through at that point, yet there he was, alive and more or less well. He didn't have multiple myeloma, but he did have a similar cancer. If he could survive, why couldn't I?

One of my biggest fears when I got sick was that my illness would cause my anxiety attacks to worsen. In fact, the opposite happened. Within months of being told I had cancer, my panic attacks began to disappear. And within a year, for the first time since I had been a sophomore in high school, they were all but gone. I can't explain it myself, and neither could Dr. Gol, but that was what happened. Not that I recommend it as a cure, and not that I didn't have new anxieties to contend with, but a real, immediate worry seemed to chase away, or at least crowd out, my vague, more distant ones. Therapy helped my cancer, but cancer also helped my therapy.

3.

AFTER I GOT sick, a number of people asked me if I was going to quit my job, if my priorities had perhaps shifted. They wanted to know if I planned to spend less time working and more time with Didi and A.J. or my family and friends. To be honest, the answer was no.

Earlier in my career, I used to fantasize about changing professions. After a bad day, or sometimes for no particular reason, I would imagine what it would be like to move to Wyoming and become a fishing guide or go to culinary school in Paris or teach. But after I got sick, I rarely thought about that. I took the same long, hard look at my work life that many people who experience a serious medical diagnosis or another seismic life event do, but instead of discovering some alternative true calling, I decided I liked what I was doing. I found my work challenging and rewarding. To the extent that what I did helped inform and entertain people, and maybe even occasionally right a wrong, it made me feel useful. I loved the process of dreaming up story ideas, finding the right writers to pursue them, and working with photographers and designers to bring them to life. It was a thrill to create something out of nothing every week. Adam was a wonderful editor whom I was learning a great deal from, and I liked and admired many of my colleagues. Instead of leading me to quit my job, getting sick helped me see how valuable it is to have work you enjoy and how lucky I was to have it.

Work was also a welcome distraction. The busier I was, the less time I had to think about cancer. A few friends or family members worried that working too hard might exacerbate my illness, but there is good stress and bad stress. My job was demanding, but I liked it. It wasn't stressful to me. Working at a job I didn't like or being home and bored would have been stressful.

I did want to spend as much time as I could with my family and friends, but I wanted to do that alongside my work, not in place of it. Besides, I was in remission and feeling fine. There was no reason for me not to work.

Even if I'd wanted to chuck it all, that wouldn't have been feasible. One of the challenges of living with a long-term incurable illness is that you need to support yourself for many years even while your ability to work may be compromised. Didi and I were both fortunate enough to have good jobs, but living in New York is expensive, and if I had stopped working, we would have had to move. Because we loved New York and because I needed to be near a major medical center, where the cost of living wasn't likely to be a great deal cheaper, relocating didn't make sense. All of which meant I needed a paycheck.

I also needed medical insurance. Over the past twenty years, the total cost of my healthcare expenses has run into the millions of dollars. In 2023 alone, when I would undergo the most extensive treatment I'd had to date, that figure was more than $2.6 million. Without insurance, Didi and I would be in dire financial straits.

Even though we could have gone on Didi's insurance plan, having healthcare coverage was too important for us to risk that. Now that I was sick, insurance was the foundation on which our entire financial house rested. We had deductibles to meet and copays to pay, but we could afford those. What we couldn't afford was life without insurance. If we both worked, we had my plan with Didi's plan as a backup, a belt and suspenders.

The magazine business, meanwhile, was taking on water. Advertising revenue, the lifeblood of the industry, was rushing away from magazines and onto the internet at hyperspeed. At just about every publication, budgets were being cut and people were being laid off. At one point, working in the same business had seemed romantic to me and Didi. We spoke the same work language, knew many of the same people, and went to the same parties. Now it felt as though we were passengers in the same sinking boat.

What if I lose my job? What if I lose my insurance? At one point or another, just about everyone lies awake at night worrying about these questions. When you have a chronic, incurable illness and you and your spouse are in a collapsing industry, these fears have a sharper edge.

4.

FROM THE BEGINNING of our relationship, Didi and I have generally split our domestic responsibilities fifty-fifty. Whereas I do the cooking, she does the cleaning. Whereas I manage the finances, she handles our social life. After A.J. was born, we took turns feeding her, changing her diapers, and putting her to sleep.

After I got sick, Didi occasionally had to pick up the slack if I had an appointment or treatment, but as much as we could, we stuck to our precancer routines. I had no physical reason not to do that, I didn't want to burden Didi if I could help it, and keeping busy helped me keep my mind off of my illness.

That's also just who we were. Perhaps to a fault, Didi and I both have a strong independent streak. For her, that likely traces back to losing her father at such a young age. For me, it may have to do with being the last of four children. In either instance, we picked up the same message: You'd better learn to fend for yourself. Neither of us likes to feel dependent on someone else.

Our desire to maintain a sense of normalcy also applied to our social life. We took A.J. to visit my parents and siblings and mother-in-law, and they came to visit us, just as we had done before. I went out to bars with friends and played in a weekly poker game. Didi had friends and colleagues over for dinner and attended a book group. We went to the movies and out to dinner with other couples.

In a well-known 1978 essay titled "Illness as Metaphor," the writer and critic Susan Sontag wrote, "Illness is the night-side of life, a more onerous citizenship. Everyone who is born holds dual citizenship, in the kingdom of the well and in the kingdom of the sick." When I was diagnosed, a crack opened between my life before cancer and my life after it, between those two realms. Maintaining a sense of normalcy at work, at home, and everywhere else helped me and Didi keep from crossing over.

5.

IN THE SUMMER of 1998, Didi and I had taken a trip to Jackson, Wyoming. Early in our relationship, we had established a pattern of alternating between vacation spots—big cities (Didi's preference) and outdoorsy destinations (mine)—and it was my turn to pick. I chose Jackson because it is a big enough town in its own right, with good restaurants, charming lodges and hotels, and cute shops, but is also smack in the middle of some of the most spectacular wilderness areas in the world, with Grand Teton and Yellowstone national parks close by.

Didi and I spent the first four or five days hiking, biking, and sightseeing; then one night we asked the desk clerk at the inn where we were staying what else she might recommend we do. "Have you tried fly-fishing?" she asked.

Neither of us had, but each of us had fished in the conventional manner as kids, me with my father and grandfather, Didi with her father, and we were intrigued by fly-fishing. The movie version of *A River Runs Through It,* Norman Maclean's semiautobiographical 1976 novella about family, loss, and fly-fishing directed by Robert Redford and starring a young Brad Pitt, had been released in 1992, and the craze for the sport that the film had sparked was still in the air. We decided to try it.

The desk clerk booked us a guide, and at 7:00 A.M. the next day, a young and friendly Jackson native named Tim Warren pulled up in his pickup truck, drift boat in tow. By 8:00 A.M., we were standing on a bank of the Snake River, with Tim giving us casting lessons. By 9:00, we had slid the boat into the water and were headed downstream.

The stretch of water we fished that day is one of the prettiest in the world, an aqueous ribbon of clean, clear emerald green winding through stands of cottonwood and aspen trees beneath the shadow of the 13,775-foot, glacier-capped Grand Teton mountain. It's not uncommon to see bald eagles, moose, and other wildlife as you make your way along.

I was fishing in the front of the boat, and Didi in the back, with Tim rowing in the middle. Somewhere around 10:30 A.M., I heard a shout. Didi had caught her first fish on a fly. Not long after, I landed mine. They were both wild, native Yellowstone cutthroats, a species famed for the distinctive bright orange slashes, or "cuts," on their throats. Neither of them was anything to speak of, size-wise, but to us they were whoppers. We took pictures of our catches and released them. In the pictures, we look like we just struck gold.

We went on to catch maybe a dozen more fish that day (in keeping with the sport's general practice, we released everything we caught), and afterward Didi, Tim, and I had dinner at a restaurant with an outdoor patio that had views of the river and mountains. Tim's girlfriend met us, too, and the four of us ate and drank and talked and laughed and watched the sun go down over the Tetons. It was a magical day and the beginning of a lifelong friendship with Tim.

From that time on, fly-fishing became an abiding passion of mine. I started taking trips to Wyoming, Idaho, the Bahamas, and other fishy spots as often as I could. I devoured books and videos about the sport. I spent weekends practicing my casting. To help finance my habit, I began writing about fishing as a side gig.

In every way, I was hooked.

For a time, the sport was an enjoyable diversion. But after my diagnosis, it became more like a necessity, as vital to my well-being as oxygen or water. Fishing may not be my church (again, I don't practice my religion) or my therapy (I had Dr. Gol for that), but I began to use it for similar purposes.

Like certain other pursuits—yoga, meditation, knitting—

fly-fishing has a Zen quality to it. The concentration required is all-consuming. When you stare at a tiny imitation insect floating on the surface of the water twenty or thirty feet from you and devote every ounce of your consciousness to the possibility that a creature might appear out of the depths at any moment to devour it, your brain doesn't have a chance to wander to work problems, money troubles, or illness. All the chatter that normally clutters your mind disappears. You are fully present, or "in the zone."

The late Dr. Herbert Benson, the founder of the pioneering Benson-Henry Institute for Mind Body Medicine at Massachusetts General Hospital in Boston and a professor at Harvard Medical School, talked about the connection between fly-fishing and the brain in a 2015 Harvard Medical School publication.

Over the millennia, Benson was quoted as saying, humans have learned various ways to turn off stress by disrupting their normal thought patterns. "What better example of this than fly-fishing," he said, "with the repetitive back-and-forth motion of the rod and line and fly? You're focusing on where that fly is going to land on the water and that breaks the train of everyday thought."

The article cited research indicating that among Americans hoping to take up fly-fishing and other forms of angling, 38 percent see fishing as a means to relax and relieve stress. "Many of these prospective anglers think the soothing sound of flowing water and the pull of a fishing line would be enough to drive their stress away," the article reported.

The article also referred to the "fight-or-flight" mechanism, or "stress response." Although that response is a useful adaptation for dealing with short-term threats, the story noted, "the modern stressful situations of unemployment, financial distress, divorce, or chronic illness, can also be permanently damaging." If stress hormone levels are elevated over time, Benson said, they can damage our immune systems, making us more vulnerable to everything from infections and illnesses to memory loss.

In 1975, Benson coined the term *relaxation response* (and wrote a book by the same name) to describe a mechanism that counteracts the stress response. Brought on by activities that induce a state of deep rest, the relaxation response changes our reactions to stress, slowing down our breathing rates, relaxing our muscles, and reducing our blood pressure.

The Harvard article noted that a 2008 study by the Benson-Henry Institute, published in *The Journal of Alternative and Complementary Medicine,* "found that more than half of the study participants who practiced the relaxation response experienced a drop in blood pressure after eight weeks, and 50 percent of those who practiced the technique were able to have their dosages of blood pressure medication lowered.

"With its meditative-like repetitive motion," the article continued, "Benson says fly-fishing is a 'beautiful way' of evoking the relaxation response."

The article went on to cite a 2009 study of combat veterans conducted by a team of researchers from the University of Southern Maine, the University of Utah, and the Department of Veterans Affairs in Salt Lake City. Participants in the study, the researchers reported, "had significant reductions in stress and post-traumatic stress disorder symptoms and improvements in sleep quality after participating in a fly-fishing retreat." (Similar programs exist for fly-fishers with cancer.)

The article concluded by noting that fly-fishing has been compared to meditation, in that fly-fishers perform a simple, repeated task, often for significant periods of time. "The motion of fly-fishing is part and parcel of the activity itself and may contribute to its calming effect," Benson noted. "Besides, it's achieving something—you might catch a fish!"

Fly-fishing's therapeutic appeal is only one of its charms. Every cast is its own tiny story, with its own potential for success and failure, tension and resolution, joy and sorrow— a dramatic miniature of life that you can play out over and over again, as often as you like. And the excitement of catching a fish never gets old. *Did that really just happen? Was I somehow able to coax that wild creature onto my line?*

Because trout thrive in cold, fast water, they're generally found in high-mountain streams. And popular saltwater species to catch on a fly, such as bonefish and tarpon, live on vast, tropical, white sand flats. In a sense, the sport is just an excuse to travel to some of the world's most remote and beautiful places.

The fish themselves are similarly stunning. The markings of a rainbow trout are every bit as magical as the phenomenon for which the species is named. Brown trout, with their multicolored spots arranged in infinite variegated patterns, are living works of Abstract Expressionism. The copper-colored "cuts" on the underside of a cutthroat trout's jaw are a shade of orange so entirely natural, so elementally outdoorsy, it's hard to get it out of your head once you've seen it.

You could spend lifetimes studying how, when, and why fish feed. Water temperature, depth, and speed are factors. So are air temperature, sun, clouds, rain, and barometric pressure. The time of day matters, as do the time of year and the moon phase. It's a beautiful, bottomless mystery.

Anglers obsess over which flies to fish at what place and at what time like rabbinical scholars study the Talmud. If the fish were eating a size 16 woolly bugger yesterday, why aren't they eating it today? What if I trim the wings on that salmon fly a bit? Or color its abdomen with a brown Sharpie? Will that make it look more natural?

Even when you're not casting to fish, just witnessing them emerge from the watery darkness and feed on natural flies is captivating. I once googled "Fish eating flies," and the search engine returned more than 24 million results.

There's an old joke: "Fishing is a jerk on one end of a line waiting for a jerk on the other." That's true enough, but a large part of the appeal of fly-fishing is that it requires a certain degree of skill. Casting a fly line is an experiment in applied physics, with dozens of moving parts, that demands coordination, precise timing, the proper application of power and finesse, and all manner of other things that are all too easy to make a hash out of. Presenting your fly so it looks natural, setting the hook on time when a fish strikes, and landing fish also take time to learn. Depending on the situation and conditions, a beginner may well catch fish, but fly-fishing is an undertaking that generally requires commitment, patience, and effort to master. When you feel that jerk on the other end of your line, you don't just feel lucky; you feel that you've accomplished something.

When you get sick, you realize how valuable it is to find something in your life that is unfailingly enjoyable, something that reliably takes your mind off your difficulties, whatever they may be. On the water, I had found such a refuge.

"One great thing about fly fishing," Norman Maclean wrote in *A River Runs Through It*, "is that after a while nothing exists of the world but thoughts about fly fishing."

6.

ALL STRESS IS hard on people, but research shows that uncertainty is difficult to deal with in unique ways.

Kate Sweeny is a psychology professor at the University of California, Riverside, who studies so-called high-stakes waiting periods and how people respond to them. Over the years, she has studied various groups while they waited for information in high-stress situations, from law school students awaiting bar exam scores to women waiting for breast biopsy results.

In an effort to better understand uncertainty, I reached out to her by Zoom. Sweeny has a bright smile and wavy blond hair. She is quick-minded and empathetic. The first thing she said to me was "I imagine you know more about the things I study than you'd like to."

As an undergraduate psychology major at Furman University in Greenville, South Carolina, Sweeny attended a lecture by a visiting professor from the University of Florida about bracing for the worst, the tendency people have to become more pessimistic as they get closer to a moment of truth, such as getting back the results of a medical test. Sweeny found the concept relatable and counterintuitive. "It's in contrast to the general human tendency to be optimistic about our own outcomes," she told me.

In graduate school, she studied bracing for the worst and related topics, such as how to give bad news and doctor-patient communication. When she finished her PhD and began looking for teaching positions, she found that she was "a nervous wreck" while she was waiting to hear if she'd gotten a job. "It wasn't life or death, but it felt like it," she said. "I was kind of a basket case."

When she got her position at UC Riverside, she decided to make high-stakes waiting the focus of her work. Her personal experience with the phenomenon inspired her, as did the fact that her mother had had non-Hodgkin's lymphoma when Sweeny was younger. "The oddities and uncertainties around that motivated me," she said. "It's fascinating how these things can get buried deep inside of us, then show up years later."

She also found that high-stakes waiting was poorly understood and not well studied. "When I would bring it up with people, they would say, 'Well, it's just stress, right? It's just coping.' That's true to an extent," she said, "but there's also something unique about this kind of stress to the point where people will say, 'I'd rather have the bad thing happen than continue to wait.'"

In one study Sweeny led, fifty law students who were preparing for the California bar exam answered questionnaires at six separate points in time: shortly before and after the exam, at two time points during the four-month waiting period before learning if they had passed, and immediately before and after learning whether they had passed. Among the study's conclusions: Waiting is more difficult at the start and end of a waiting period. "It's a U-shaped curve," she said. "You worry a lot at the beginning, sort of forget about it in the middle, then worry a lot again at the end."

But her most notable conclusion was that even when the students received bad news, they were relieved to get it. "If they failed, they didn't feel good," she said. "But that anxiety just went away. The waiting really is the hardest part."

Sweeny has also studied coping techniques for uncertainty. In 2019, she and fellow researchers investigated whether "flow," or being fully absorbed in an activity, helped people in three anxiety-inducing situations: law school graduates waiting for their bar exam results, doctorate-level students in the academic job market awaiting matches to internships and residencies, and undergraduates waiting for peers to rate their physical attractiveness. Participating in flow-inducing activities, they found, boosts people's sense of well-being during a period of uncertainty and makes the waiting a little easier.

In 2020, Sweeny and other researchers collaborated with scientists from Central China Normal University in Wuhan to study the impact of flow on long periods of quarantine. More than five thousand participants in Wuhan and other major cities in China affected by covid completed an online survey in which they assessed the length of their quarantine, their overall well-being during the past week, and any flow activities they had experienced during the same period.

The researchers found that people in a lengthy quarantine who reported a higher-than-average number of flow experiences were no worse off in terms of overall wellness than people who had not yet quarantined. Engaging in flow-inducing activities such as running, painting, and gardening seemed to protect against the potentially harmful effects of quarantine.

The lack of control people typically feel in high-stakes waiting situations is also anxiety-inducing, Sweeny has found. "Not only do you not know what's coming, but you can't do anything about it."

Worry can be a useful alarm bell, she said. "Those of us who had it probably survived longer than those who didn't." That's helpful when you can do something about your fears—if you're worried about getting in a car accident, you can buy a safer car or wear your seat belt.

But when you're waiting for a bar exam result or a biopsy, there's not much you can do. "You basically have an alarm bell that's stuck in the on position and can't be turned off. When there's no job for worry to do, it can be damaging." Exerting control however they can seems to give people some relief, Sweeny said. Participants in her studies have reported doing things such as getting more familiar with their medical insurance policy, researching the best doctor to see, and investigating what clinical trials are available, even before they receive a diagnosis. "All in all, doing something is better than doing nothing."

It can also be helpful to look for silver linings in bad news before it actually arrives. Sweeny calls that "preemptive benefit finding" or "predemption." "We know people do this after they've experienced bad news, trauma, and grief. But it turns out it can be helpful *before* getting bad news, too."

In one study, Sweeny asked people undergoing a breast biopsy, "Is there any good you can imagine that might come out of it if you find out you have breast cancer?"

"I thought maybe it would be insulting to even ask, but roughly three-quarters of the participants said, 'Absolutely. I would appreciate my family more. I'd be a role model for my daughters. I'd get healthier.' That sort of thing. Our evidence shows it helps people cope if they've already thought that through."

Social support is helpful in any stressful situation, including uncertainty instances, she said. "Epidemiological studies have found that a lack of support may be more predictive of what we call all-cause mortality, or mortality with all factors accounted for, than something like smoking."

At the same time, offering and receiving support are hard to do well, Sweeny said, particularly in uncertainty situations, in which neither party knows exactly what they're facing. "People experiencing uncertainty don't always know what they want," she said. "If they ask for help, it can make them feel needy or weak. If they get it, it doesn't always make them feel better." As a support partner, "it's surprisingly challenging to get it right." What's the best way to be helpful? Do you call? Do you not? Do you buy a gift? Do you send food? "The research is basically all over the map. No one thing really works. And if you don't get it right, you feel guilty and frustrated."

The breakthrough research on the subject, Sweeny said, was done by Harry Reis, a psychology professor at the University of Rochester, and expanded on by Shelly Gable, a social psychologist at the University of California, Santa Barbara. The key is something called perceived responsiveness, meaning whether the person *feels* supported. That sense appears to come from three factors: Does the person feel understood ("I get it, I hear you"), valued ("I love you"), and cared for ("I'm here to help")? "It's the idea that 'Maybe X, Y, or Z wasn't the perfect thing to do, but I know the person meant well and that's actually all that matters,'" Sweeny said. You still have to figure out how to communicate that you care, she says, whether that's by what you say or just by showing up to sit with someone. "But if it's clear you understand, value, and care about someone, almost anything you do can be helpful."

For all the insights she's gained, Sweeny is still surprised—and troubled—by one overarching fact: "None of the coping mechanisms people use are really very effective." Even she, after all the research she's done, has difficulty managing her anxieties. When she's worried about something, she said, people sometimes ask her, "You've studied this. Aren't you better at it?" "I'm afraid the answer is 'No, I'm really not,'" she said. "I still get very worried about things. Worry is hard to drive away."

She takes comfort in the fact that techniques such as flow and "predemption" can help to some degree. "Your worries will still be waiting for you when you're done, but you can at least get a few hours of rest, which is valuable." If nothing else, it can be useful to know you're not alone. "If coping with uncertainty seems hard, it helps to know that's normal."

7.

CATHERINE SANDERSON IS a psychology professor at Amherst College, my alma mater (she began teaching there after I graduated). In addition to her academic work, Sanderson writes books, newspaper stories, and magazine articles that translate psychological research into everyday language for general audiences, with an eye toward improving public health, and I've worked with her as an editor.

In researching the subject of uncertainty, I e-mailed Sanderson for advice on finding experts on the topic, and it turned out she had written about it herself. During the covid pandemic, with rates of anxiety, depression, and other mental health disorders skyrocketing, she realized that it wasn't just the coronavirus that was ubiquitous, but "there was a parallel epidemic of uncertainty. And it wasn't just cancer patients or other people in special situations who were experiencing it," she told me. "It was all of us." In an attempt to help people experiencing those problems, she surveyed the literature on the science of uncertainty and wrote an article titled "The Psychology of Understanding and Managing Uncertainty" for *Psychology Today*.

To discuss the subject further, I talked to Sanderson by video chat as well. A self-described "psychology nerd," she speaks at New York speed and has a palpable enthusiasm for her work.

Psychologists make a distinction between acute stress and chronic stress, she told me. "Acute stress is 'I broke my ankle,' and chronic stress is 'I'm living in poverty and I'm constantly

worried about if my kids are going to have enough to eat."
While the human fight-or-flight response is useful for coping
with acute stress, she said, it's not helpful when it comes to
chronic stress. "It keeps us at a high level of arousal for prolonged periods of time, which can cause problems ranging
from anxiety to compromised immunity."

To illustrate just how difficult it is for people to deal with
uncertainty, she pointed to research in her *Psychology Today*
story showing that "people who have a 50% chance of receiving an electric shock feel more stress than people who
have a 100% chance of receiving a shock." "It's a fascinating
finding," she said. "People are basically saying the anticipation of pain feels worse than the pain itself."

When we spoke, Sanderson was teaching a seminar on
close relationships and had come across research showing
that people who are widowed experience lower rates of premature death than people who are divorced. "That might
seem odd," she said, "in that people who are widowed have
lost somebody, whereas people who are divorced know their
former partner is still alive and out there, they're just no longer married to them." But being divorced involves exactly
the sort of ongoing uncertainty that's difficult for people to
deal with, she said. "People who are divorced often ask
themselves endless questions: 'Could we someday get back
together? Is this person going to get married again? Are we
going to have a conflict about child support?'"

That stress, Sanderson said, can have unique effects.
"Being widowed is a devastating event for people, but at least
there's a finality to it. You're not wondering 'Is this person
going to be alive again?' There's a sense of closure."

The detrimental effects of uncertainty are so powerful
that people who report persistent concern about losing their
jobs experience worse health and higher rates of depression

than people who get fired, Sanderson noted in her *Psychology Today* story. She cited research indicating that "chronic job insecurity is a stronger predictor of poor health than smoking or high blood pressure."

To illustrate how powerful a pull uncertainty can have on our thoughts, she cited a study in which college women were given information about how a male student felt about them. "Some were told the male student liked them a lot, others were told he liked them an average amount, and still others were told the man either liked them a lot or an average amount (the uncertainty condition)," she wrote.

Whom did the women find the most attractive? "Not surprisingly, women were more attracted to the men who liked them a lot than the men who liked them an average amount," she wrote. "But they were most attracted to—and found themselves thinking about the most—the men in the uncertain condition."

When we're unsure if someone likes us, it occupies our attention, she told me. "We can't stop wondering 'Does she like me, or doesn't she?' We have a need to keep mulling it over." When we know someone doesn't like us, there may be a sense of rejection, but there is, again, finality. "There's the old *Sex and the City* line," she said. " 'He's just not that into you.' " As blunt as that sentiment is, she said, it can be useful. "It's like ripping the Band-Aid off. It hurts for a moment, but then it's over."

Chronic uncertainty is also difficult to deal with because it inhibits our ability to act, leaving us in a suspended waiting game, Sanderson told me. In her *Psychology Today* article, she quoted a passage from the Alan Paton novel *Cry, the Beloved Country:* "Sorrow is better than fear. Fear is a journey, a terrible journey, but sorrow is at least an arrival."

"Have you heard about fight, flight, or freeze?" she asked me.

I hadn't, I told her.

"It's like fight or flight 2.0," she said. "In psychology, we now talk about three responses when we face a threat: We fight, we run, or we become paralyzed." Paralysis is particularly insidious, she said. "Not only does it not solve the problem, but it can create the sense that the problem *can't* be solved, which can make us feel helpless."

In terms of coping with uncertainty, Sanderson suggested three strategies: Control what you can control, and make peace with what you can't; distract yourself from negative thoughts (flow activities are ideal, she said, but simpler diversions can also help); and reach out to others.

The previous year, she told me, her husband had lost his job. It was a position he had held for more than twenty years, and he had been let go suddenly and unfairly, she said. "We were definitely facing uncertainty." At first, she and her husband were reluctant to share what had happened with anyone except a few family members and close friends. They felt isolated and alone. But when they eventually started telling more people what happened, they felt "flooded with love and support." In some ways, they "never felt more loved."

"In psychology, we talk about two different kinds of support, problem focused and emotional," she said. "The first is 'Oh, you have cancer? I know a great doctor.' The second is 'I'm sorry. I understand. I know you're scared and worried, and I'm here for you.' " Her comments brought to mind the idea of perceived responsiveness that Kate Sweeny had mentioned and the value of making a person feel understood, valued, and cared for.

When someone is facing uncertainty, Sanderson told me,

practical support can be helpful, but basic sympathy and compassion can be every bit as powerful, if not more so. "What we know about stress in general is it's made better by feeling like you're not alone. When people are experiencing uncertainty and they feel they have to cope with it on their own, that alone can make it worse."

8.

I WASN'T AWARE of Kate Sweeny or Catherine Sanderson in the days and months following my diagnosis, but it turns out that my experience of coping with uncertainty was eerily consistent with their findings. Waiting was more difficult for me at the beginning and end of a waiting period. When I got bad news, it was better, in some ways, than not knowing; at least it relieved the torture of waiting. Bracing for the worst ahead of time helped me accept upsetting information when it did come, as did distracting myself and looking for silver linings. Any support I received from loved ones, overt or perceived, practical or emotional, was a balm.

I can't say that any of that was by design. I lucked into having Dr. Gol to consult with, I am fortunate to have friends and family who care about me, and I stumbled into most of my other strategies, if you can call them that. But somehow, however haphazardly, I was learning to live with my illness and the myriad worries it brought.

Still, and also consistent with Sweeny's research, nothing I did ultimately made my fears go away. Living with an incurable disease, I found, was basically like waiting for a bar exam or biopsy result forever. Although I was no longer having acute anxiety attacks, I had permanent, low-key anxiety to contend with.

Do you recall the myth of Damocles? He was an ancient

Greek who envied his king, Dionysius, for his wealth and power. Dionysius agreed to trade places with Damocles for a day, allowing Damocles to sit on his throne, but then hung a sword over his head to represent the dangers and anxieties that wealth and power bring.

Beginning immediately after my remission and continuing in the years since, no matter how many hours I've spent on Dr. Gol's couch, no matter how busy I've kept myself with work, no matter how fortunate I am to have medical insurance and the financial resources not to go bankrupt, no matter how many trout streams I've stood in, no matter how much emotional support I enjoy, no matter how many uncertainty researchers I've spoken to, that's how I've felt: To one degree or another, I am constantly aware of the threat that hangs over me.

I am Damocles, and cancer is my sword.

9.

ON SUNDAY, APRIL 18, 2004, two days after I was pronounced cancer free, Didi went to pick up a grocery bag, and— *Zing!*—a jolt of pain shot down her spine. That night, she woke me up at two. She was crying. She couldn't move. We called 911, and the paramedics took her to the emergency room, where a doctor gave her painkillers and muscle relaxers and diagnosed her with bulging L5 and L6 discs. She had never had back problems before. Could you read this as an instance of a woman who had been carrying too heavy a load for too long and finally cracked because she could? Yes, you could.

Caregiver burden, also known as caregiver burnout, refers to the ways in which caring for another individual—say, an elderly person or someone who is seriously ill—can weigh on the caregiver. Allison Applebaum is an authority on the subject.

A clinical psychologist specializing in psycho-oncology and the author of *Stand by Me: A Guide to Navigating Modern, Meaningful Caregiving,* Applebaum was working as a postdoctoral fellow at Memorial Sloan Kettering Cancer Center in 2010, providing care to patients in advanced stages of the disease, when she was asked to think about how Sloan Kettering could improve its psycho-oncology care and what areas of her field had not yet been fully explored.

As numerous patients told her about their caregivers and how much they worried about the effects of caregiving, Applebaum came to realize how important caregivers are, how taxing their role can be, and how little support is available for them.

The following year, in 2011, Applebaum founded the Caregivers Clinic at Sloan Kettering. The clinic's mission is to provide the caregivers of cancer patients with resources and support for everything from coping with the shock of a patient's diagnosis to dealing with their loss.

The same year Applebaum founded the Caregivers Clinic, she became a caregiver herself. After experiencing heart and kidney problems for several years, Applebaum's father, Stanley, was diagnosed in 2013 with Lewy body disease, a progressive neurodegenerative condition. (Stanley Applebaum was a well-known composer and arranger who had worked on Ben E. King's "Stand by Me"—hence the title of Applebaum's book.) Post-diagnosis, Applebaum began serving as a caregiver for Stanley, and after her mother passed away in 2014, Applebaum became her father's primary caregiver, remaining so until his death in 2019.

To learn more about caregiver burden, I spoke to Applebaum, again by video call, from her office at Sloan Kettering.

With long brown hair and blue-green eyes, Applebaum is equal parts warm and professional. She exhibits the kind of dedication to her work that's often inspired by personal experience.

At the time we spoke, Applebaum told me, some 53 million Americans identified as caregivers, with most assisting parents or children and many taking care of spouses or partners. Almost half of caregivers provide care to older people and nearly two-thirds to people with long-term health problems, she said. The average time caregivers spend in that role is four and a half years, with many doing so for more than ten years. And caregivers devote an average of twenty-five hours per week to tending to the needs of others, she said, with many spending more than forty-one hours per week— the equivalent of a full-time job.

The assistance caregivers provide, she told me, ranges from helping with everyday tasks, such as shopping, housework, and managing finances to aiding their charges with daily living issues, such as getting dressed, showering, and using the bathroom, to performing medical and nursing procedures, such as taking blood pressure readings, changing bandages, or administering injections. Two-thirds of caregivers, she said, carry out their role while holding down a paying job.

Across all age groups, caregiving is associated with an array of physical and mental health problems, Applebaum told me, including anxiety, depression, and post-traumatic stress disorder. PTSD is a particular focus of her research. When we spoke, she was conducting a study about PTSD among survivors of stem cell transplantation. Early in the study, as she had been attempting to recruit participants, she had had trouble finding a sufficient number of people who met the required diagnostic criteria for PTSD, she said. But when she opened the study to the caregivers of transplant survivors, she found that nearly 80 percent of them met the criteria. (She later submitted a grant to the National Institutes of Health to replicate the whole trial in caregivers.) "What that tells us," she told me, "is that there is a large population of caregivers in this country walking around with untreated aftereffects."

Like veterans of war and other trauma survivors, caregivers are frequently exposed to situations involving extreme emotional intensity, from receiving news about a diagnosis to taking their charges to the emergency room or witnessing their death, she told me. As a result, caregivers may experience intrusive memories from those events, hypersensitivity to the idea that something may go wrong, and irritability.

As caregiving consumes significant amounts of their time and resources, many caregivers experience sadness, fear, anxiety, and feelings of isolation. Those who are forced to put career, family, or other goals aside may also feel resentment, particularly if they feel they had no choice in taking on that role or have a difficult relationship with the person they're caring for. "That can lead to anger about not being able to plan their life, opportunities lost, and dreams deferred."

Guilt can also enter the equation, she told me. No matter how much caregivers do, they often feel that they're not doing enough or that they're not entitled to their own feelings. Some feel especially guilty when they take the time to take care of their own needs.

Romantic couples in which one partner becomes the caregiver for the other often face unique issues. "There's a shift in roles. Many caregivers struggle to remain connected to the romantic part while they're actively taking care of their partner." Romantic partners are also often partners in life, partners in a home, and partners in day-to-day obligations, she said. When one partner is sick, the other often has to take on added responsibilities. "That can lead to resentment, too."

In Applebaum's practice, she has seen illness and caregiving in romantic couples generally lead to one of two outcomes. In one case, "the relationship wasn't that strong to begin with. The illness comes in, there's a breakdown in communication, and the relationship doesn't survive." In the other, the illness and caregiving strengthen the partnership. "This is usually in the couples who have good communication skills and are able to put those skills to work."

Physically, caregiver burden has been shown to cause issues including high blood pressure, heart disease, decreased immunity, and fatigue. In *Stand by Me,* Applebaum cited a Swedish study of almost three hundred thousand spousal caregivers of cancer patients. The study, she wrote, found that caregivers had "increased risks of coronary heart disease and stroke that persisted over time, and that such risks were particularly high among caregivers of patients with cancers with high mortality rates, like pancreatic, liver, and lung cancers." She also cited a study of more than 1,500 caregivers of cancer survivors in the United States who had been followed for eight years. Those researchers, she wrote, "identified high rates of heart disease, arthritis, and chronic back pain several years after initial caregiving experiences."

The demands of caregiving may also lead people to neglect their own health and wellness, she told me. "While caregivers are phenomenal at taking care of others, they don't always prioritize their own needs."

Although caregivers are not typically compensated for the work they do, they often incur additional expenses that can include the direct costs of medical treatment, the increased sharing of household expenses, or a loss of income. One large study of the direct cost of cancer care alone, Apple-baum wrote in *Stand by Me,* found that patients and their caregivers spend between $180 and $2,600 each month on that care.

Juggling multiple caregiving roles is another challenge many caregivers face, Applebaum said. An estimated 9 million Americans are "sandwich generation" caregivers, providing care for both children and adults, and studies show that caregivers who attend to more than one generation at a time have more health problems and are less likely to seek treatment than those who provide care to one adult.

Oddly enough, caregivers often experience problems just as the individuals they're caring for get better, Applebaum told me. "It's often the first time they can take a step back, look at what just happened, and exhale. All the emotions they've been holding in check come rushing to the surface." When I told her what had happened with Didi's back, she said she has seen many instances like it.

The most effective way for caregivers to cope with caregiver burden, she said, is to ask for help. Even if only they can manage the primary caregiving responsibilities, they may be able to delegate certain tasks, such as grocery shopping or managing finances. She also recommends support groups, which can help caregivers "feel less alone and more 'normal.'"

Taking time to appreciate the positive aspects of caregiving can also be helpful, Applebaum told me. Finding meaning in caregiving, in fact, is another focus of her research. That process can take different forms for different people. "Some people have told me, 'I didn't know how strong or capable I was until I cared for someone else.' Others have said, 'I used to be shy, but because I've had to speak up with all these physicians, I've learned to find my voice.'" Still other caregivers realize they have a passion for the work and change careers to something related.

Although Applebaum would undo her father's illness and death in an instant if she could—"He was my best friend," she told me—she is nonetheless grateful for the lessons that caring for him taught her. While she is quick to point out that she doesn't mean to minimize the difficulties of caregiving, she appreciates its gifts. "Like so many caregivers," she wrote in *Stand by Me*, "I have emerged from years of living with intense uncertainty as a much stronger, more confident, grounded, and peaceful version of myself."

10.

DIDI HAS EXPERIENCED many of the effects of caregiver burden. After the incident with her bulging discs, her back problems became chronic. The smallest misstep or awkward twist could cause days of pain. Sometimes stress alone seemed to be the culprit. More than once her back trouble flared when I was due to be retested or after I received bad medical news.

After I was diagnosed, Didi also began to get migraine headaches, sometimes sporadically, other times as often as once a week. At times, they were so bad that she would have to lie in bed with the lights off and a cold washcloth on her forehead or go to the emergency room for IV morphine. Her neurologist told her that migraines might have been caused by family history (migraines are often hereditary), hormonal changes brought on by childbirth, the stress of my diagnosis, or all of the above.

Although my diagnosis didn't change the way Didi and I divided our practical responsibilities with A.J. or around the house, my illness saddled Didi with added emotional burdens. She was the person who took on the responsibility of answering questions from family and friends about how I was doing and keeping them informed about what was going on with me. And the prospect of potentially having to raise A.J. as a single parent loomed. At the time, Didi said that the possibility didn't worry her because she didn't believe I would die from cancer. I appreciated the optimism, and I think she genuinely felt that way. But later she came to realize that the thought was, at least in part, a form of denial.

Didi also had to put up with my moods. Although I wasn't clinically depressed or anxious, I wasn't myself, either. Some of my worst qualities—condescension, being a know-it-all, a desire to be in control—became more pronounced. I picked on her for petty things: The dishes weren't loaded the way I liked them to be or the laundry wasn't folded exactly as I preferred it.

Although Didi was often emotionally distant, she wasn't uncaring. She would ask how I was feeling and what she could do to help. If I had a test, a treatment, or an appointment, she would wish me well and sometimes accompany me. For the most part, I didn't want her to come to my treatments; it kept me calmer to know she was taking care of herself and A.J. At the same time, I wanted her to be all in on caring for me, or something close to that, anyway, and anything short of that was unacceptable.

I could also be short-tempered. At one point, Didi was concerned that I was depressed and called Dr. Gruenstein to ask for advice. Speaking to my doctor without my permission may or may not have been the right thing for her to do, and as it turned out, I wasn't depressed, just "normally upset" by my situation. But it was a well-intended gesture regardless. Still, I blew up at her. How dare she go behind my back like that?

Despite the fact that her husband had cancer, Didi felt as

though she had to be cheerful at all times. Not only was she trying to keep up my spirits, for my sake and hers, but we didn't want A.J. to pick up the feeling that anything was wrong. Didi also had to deal with the anxiety my screening tests brought. Just as I had to await the results, so did she. What's more, she felt she had to help me manage my anxiety. When she felt sad or scared or angry about my illness, she felt guilty. Given what I was going through, she didn't feel she had the right to feel sorry for herself.

When Didi was in graduate school at Northwestern, her feelings of grief over her father's death finally caught up with her. She became depressed and began seeing a therapist and taking Prozac. She lost interest in school, barely ate, and spent days at a time in bed. To one extent or another, she has suffered from depression ever since. That only made the task of being happy at all times, impossible under the best of circumstances and doubly so when your spouse has a life-threatening illness, that much more daunting.

It is an uncomfortable truth that illness isn't attractive. For a long time, I limped. I gained weight. I had radiation burns and tattoos. Radiation diarrhea is not pretty; neither is being hairless in your groin.

Illness can be symbolically off-putting, too. Consciously or otherwise, the person you wake up next to every morning and go to bed with every night is a reminder of your single worst, most hardwired fear: the fear of death.

None of that is conducive to warm feelings or romance. We had sex, but there was a coldness to it. Our love life, physical and emotional, was drained of its warmth.

On some level, Didi realized she was angry at me, or if not at me, exactly, at what I represented: another potential tragedy. As the saying goes, you marry your father, but this isn't supposed to be what it means. And then she felt guilty for feeling that way, and I felt guilty for being the cause of it. As Allison Applebaum said, cancer either tears down a marriage or makes it stronger. In our case, my illness was beginning to do the former.

As brave a face as Didi and I both put on, as much as we resolved to "fight this thing" and "go forward" and "stay positive," as hopeful as we both were that I would survive, the fact was that I had an incurable form of cancer that might well kill me. That reality made it tough for either of us to enjoy the other's company. We stopped going out. Even garden-variety conversation was loaded. "How was your day, honey?" "Great, I had another bone marrow biopsy. You?"

Even after I was declared cancer free, things didn't normalize. If anything, they got worse. By then, our unhappiness had become self-perpetuating. We were bickering all the time, with each of us blaming the other. It was as if we were both thinking, *This relationship is terrible. It must be the other person's fault.* In retrospect, it's clear that we became afraid to love each other. The closer we got, the more difficult things would be if I died. It's as if we were trying to get a jump-start on life after my death.

At one point, I told Dr. Gol I noticed I was withdrawing from A.J. My logic was that it was better for her to never know her father than to know him and later miss him. Dr. Gol said to me, "Wouldn't you rather give her as much of yourself as you can?" I was able to follow that advice with A.J., but I wasn't able to follow it with Didi, and she wasn't able to follow it with me. The tension that had built up between us was too powerful, the wall that separated us too high. Almost by the day, we grew farther apart. You know how they say you can be together with someone but still be alone? That was us.

It wasn't all bad—we had moments of returning to our precancer selves—but it was far from what either of us wanted from our marriage. Then Didi spoke up.

We were at a lodge in Jackson, Wyoming—a fishing trip plus family vacation this time—and A.J. was asleep. It started out as a conversation about a problem Didi was having at work, but somehow we found ourselves at odds, the tension started to rise, and the next thing I knew, Didi was crying and shouting. The gist of what she said was this: "This is a disaster. We are in the midst of a huge mess. I love you, but I don't like you right now. I know you don't like me, either, so don't pretend you do. What the hell are we going to do?" We shouted at each other, surfaced long-simmering resentments, and talked about getting separated or divorced.

In past relationships, that was the point at which I would check out. I would either blame the other person or pretend the issues we were having weren't a big deal. Didi wasn't going to allow that to happen. Remember what I said about Didi at our wedding: She is real. She doesn't shy away from life's difficulties. We didn't have answers to our problems at the moment, but Didi wasn't going to let us pretend they didn't exist. "I don't want to live like this," she said. "It sucks."

11.

A.J. WAS ONLY a year old when I achieved my first remission, but Didi and I had already begun wringing our hands over how and when to tell her I had cancer. Our impulse was to tell her the truth as soon as she could understand, but when would that be? And what exactly should we say? Is it right to tell a one-year-old that her father might die? Is it right to lie to her? No parent can make a guarantee to their child that they *won't* die, of course, but most can make the pledge in good faith, at least for the foreseeable future. People with an incurable, life-threatening illness can't do that.

I asked Dr. Gol what she thought we should do, and she introduced me to a concept I hadn't heard of: the need to know versus the need to tell. Didi and I had an urge to tell A.J. We wanted to be truthful with her, and we wanted the weight of the secret off of our backs. Maintaining the lie took vigilance and left us fearful that A.J. might in the coming years find out inadvertently. But at that point, A.J. didn't have a need to know. I was healthy and in no immediate danger of being otherwise. Didi and I decided to wait.

In a sense, having a young child when you find out you have cancer is awful. It feels like a particularly cruel twist of fate, and you worry, of course, about leaving them without a parent. But it's also a blessing. It's a glass of ice water thrown in your face that says, "Wake up, and spend as much time as possible with the people you love while you can."

Not only did I value the time I spent with A.J. when she was a baby more than I otherwise might have, but all the diaper changes, baths, bedtime stories, and midnight feedings that can drive other parents insane were, for me, another useful distraction. If it meant not having to go to bed and lie awake thinking about cancer, well, then, "Yes, sweetie, I would love to read you *Hop on Pop* one more time." Among a sea of troubles, A.J. was an island of happiness. I called her my little joy machine.

Multiple myeloma isn't thought to be hereditary, but my diagnosis made me paranoid about A.J.'s health, nevertheless. As a toddler, she developed a mysterious ailment in her left leg. She would try to walk on it and just fall down. None of us, not Didi or our babysitter or I, had seen her fall or otherwise hurt herself, so after a day or two, we took her to the pediatrician. The doctor recommended an X-ray, and when we got to the X-ray room, I panicked. Mysterious leg ailment? Check. MRI? No, but an X-ray was close enough.

The X-rays, of course, came back negative, and the limp disappeared as mysteriously as it had arrived. The doctor believed that it was probably a sprain that we just hadn't witnessed. Later, another theory occurred to me and Didi: A.J. had grown up with a father who had been limping for most of her life. Monkey see, monkey do.

12.

ON A SUNNY March morning in 2007, Didi and I had just walked out of our apartment, on our way to go grocery shopping. A.J., who was about to turn four, was at home with a babysitter. Didi and I had been avoiding the topic for years, out of fear about the widening cracks in our relationship and my future, but I was doing well, and after the fight we'd had in Wyoming, we had been getting along better. If nothing else, that argument had temporarily cleared the air. If we weren't exactly young newlyweds again, we weren't constantly at odds anymore, either.

That morning, with A.J. at home and out of earshot, I decided to raise the subject. After the usual chitchat about what we should get for dinner, I asked Didi, "So, should we have another kid?"

Deciding whether to bring a child into the world is a weighty question under any circumstances. But for people with an incurable illness, it's especially complicated. Is it right to bring a child into the world knowing they might have only one parent? Is it right to knowingly leave one's partner with the added burdens of single parenthood?

I started to launch into a spiel I had rehearsed in my mind

about the pros and cons of the matter. Pros: We had always said we might want to have a second child; it would be nice for A.J. to have a sibling; maybe we would have a boy to give our family "one of each." Cons: I might die prematurely, leaving two children instead of one without a father and Didi to raise both by herself. I made a point of saying that because the burden might primarily fall on Didi, she should really be the one who—

She cut me off. "Let's do it," she said.

"Really? Are you sure? I mean, you'd be the one who would have to—"

"Yes, I'm sure."

Until then, whenever I had thought of the matter, strictly theoretically, the idea had prompted a tangle of feelings: excitement, for sure, but also anxiety, fear, and guilt. But now that the possibility was real, I suddenly had a revised position. The smile that spread across my face reflected my new thinking.

Didi and I hugged outside the supermarket on University Place, then went inside to buy our Annie's mac and cheese, chicken nuggets, and Fruit Roll-Ups. When we walked down the diaper aisle, Didi said, "You know we're going to have to deal with those again, right?" Now she was the one who was smiling.

13.

ON APRIL 17, 2007, I celebrated my third anniversary cancer free and my forty-second birthday. That night, Didi and I went out to dinner, had a nice meal and some wine, and were feeling good. It was a warm spring evening, and we decided to walk home. We could have walked any number of ways, but as it happened, we walked up Broadway. It occurred to me only later that we had walked past the office where my startup was, past the spot where I had slipped on the ice.

When we got home, A.J. was asleep. We said good night to the babysitter and got ready for bed. Didi went to bed first, and I stayed up to read for a while. Later, I went into A.J.'s room. I had a pet little thing I used to say to her when I put her to bed: "I love you most of all, forever and ever, no matter what." I whispered it to her and kissed her good night.

In our bedroom, Didi was asleep. I guess it was because of the anniversary and the birthday and the beautiful night. Who knows. But what I did was, for the first time in many months, maybe a year, I took off my glasses, and I kneeled down, and when I was done, I kissed the bottom knuckles of my thumbs three times. Only this time, I didn't ask for anything or offer any bargains. I'm not sure who or what I was talking to; there were plenty of worthy subjects. Anyway, what I said was "Thank you."

T plus three years and counting.

14.

AFTER MY RADIATION therapy, I had never had my sperm count checked. I had no reason to before, but now I did.

On our first visit to the fertility clinic, Didi and I exchanged uncomfortable glances in the waiting room. Do you know how people who have been together for a long time can effectively read each other's minds? We were doing that. The source of our mutual discomfort was guilt. We already had a healthy, happy child. Many of the other couples in that room almost certainly didn't and very much wanted to. Were we being selfish for trying to conceive again? Should we count our blessings and leave well enough alone?

A few minutes later, when we shared our hesitation with

the doctor we saw, he reminded us that getting pregnant isn't a zero-sum game; we weren't denying anyone else the chance to have a baby by attempting to have one ourselves. We decided to go ahead.

As it turned out, my sperm count was on the low side of barely viable. The doctor gave us three options: try to get pregnant in the time-honored manner and see what happened, use the sperm I had frozen for artificial insemination, or use the sperm for IVF.

Because of the risks and difficulties IVF poses, we decided to try a one-two punch of old-fashioned sex and monthly insemination treatments. If those didn't work, we could still try IVF, as long as we took care not to use all my stored-up sperm in the course of the insemination.

On our doctor's advice, Didi began tracking her cycles and stopped taking birth control pills. At the appropriate time each month, we made a point of having sex and attended the fertility clinic for insemination appointments.

In case you're wondering, artificial insemination appointments are not sexy. There is a lot of sterile equipment and fluorescent lighting, and at least one of you is wearing a hospital gown. You know the old joke about the turkey baster? It's more or less true. No disrespect to anyone with a medical kink, but pipettes and cannulae are not my thing.

As part of our fertility treatment program, Didi sometimes went to the clinic without me for pregnancy tests. One morning in June, my phone rang at work, and I saw her number appear on the incoming call display. Ironically, I was working on *New York*'s "The Best Doctors" issue, and our fertility doctor was among the physicians recognized (the selections had been made by an independent research firm, not me). "Hi," I said, as dispassionately as I could.

I knew Didi had had an appointment that day, and the

previous two visits had not brought the news we were hoping for. I didn't want to be insensitive. I was also preparing myself to be disappointed.

"You won't believe this," she said, "but I'm pregnant."

She was right. I didn't believe it. It barely sounded as though she did.

If I remember correctly, my carefully measured reply was "Holy fucking shit."

That Saturday, Didi, A.J., and I went to my sister Jen's house in the suburbs for a cookout. My sister Tina was there, too. At the time, Jen lived in a condominium complex with a community pool. After lunch, we let A.J. run ahead of us to dip her feet in the water until we could catch up to watch her swim.

As the rest of us walked toward the pool, I looked at Didi as if to ask, "Now?"

She nodded yes.

"Don't scream," I said to Tina and Jen, not wanting A.J. to suspect that anything unusual was up because we hadn't told her the news yet and didn't plan to until after Didi's first trimester was over, "but Didi is pregnant."

They screamed.

PART FOUR

Recurrence

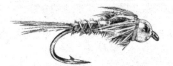

1.

ON COLUMBUS DAY 2007, I went into my office. Officially we had the day off, but I was behind in editing a true crime story about a hedge fund millionaire who had been murdered by his wife. When I finished what I was doing for the day, I hit Print, then turned around in my chair to grab the story off the printer. *Snap.* I felt something crack in my ribs.

I saw Dr. Gruenstein later that week. My ribs were sore and swollen. He ordered a CT scan, which confirmed what everyone involved suspected: I had another tumor, this one on my left tenth rib.

It had been three and a half years since I had been pronounced cancer free, a year and a half short of the five-year mark. Didi was five months pregnant.

I've been asked if it's easier to hear you have cancer the second time around. How about the third? The fourth? Do you ever get used to it?

You do, in the sense that the news is not flat-out shocking the way it is the first time and you have at least some sense of what lies ahead. But you still feel angry, anxious, and scared. No amount of context or experience ever makes the words "You have cancer" easy to hear.

The rib in question, it turned out, was comparatively easy to radiate. Once I learned that and after it was determined through the now-familiar battery of tests that I had no other lesions, I decided to have my second round of radiation treatments done not by Dr. Dalton at Mount Sinai but at St. Vincent's Hospital, near my apartment. Going to and from appointments every day for weeks is time-consuming. Once again, I was hoping to live as normal a life as possible: go to work every day, be home in the mornings and evenings with

Didi and A.J., have time to go to the gym. Being radiated close to home could help me facilitate that.

Before I could see a radiation oncologist at St. Vincent's, I needed to see a medical oncologist there to confirm my diagnosis and sign off on my treatment plan. On a cloudy November afternoon, Didi and I went to see Dr. Jagannath, the doctor I had consulted to get a second opinion about my initial diagnosis.

Once again, Dr. Jagannath confirmed my condition and endorsed the radiation plan. When I asked him if I should expect anything different this time, compared to my first round of radiation, he said no, everything should be more or less the same. But he also frankly informed me and Didi that multiple myeloma remissions tend to get shorter after each treatment. He took a pen from the pocket of his lab coat and drew a graph on the examining table tissue paper. With each incremental treatment he depicted, the distance between the remissions shrank. Then the line stopped.

Over the course of the next five weeks, I received twenty-five radiation treatments. Once again, the side effects were mild. The worst one was a burning sensation I felt up and down the right half of my body that no one could explain and after a few weeks mysteriously vanished. For all its awe-inspiring advancements, cancer treatment is still full of unknowns.

A month or so later, I underwent another battery of tests to see if the radiation had worked. The good news was that the treatment had "killed" the lesion. The bad news was that my M protein level hadn't gone back to normal (multiple myeloma can exist in your system without causing bone lesions or other overt symptoms).

Dr. Gruenstein and Dr. Jagannath agreed that the best

course of action would be watchful waiting. It was January 2008. My second child was due in a month, and I had cancer.

2.

THE EVENTS OF February 11 and 12, 2008, unfolded like an *I Love Lucy* episode.

At around 10:00 P.M. on the eleventh, Didi began having contractions, but they were mild and infrequent, and her due date was still a week away. I asked if she wanted to call the doctor, but she said no. She said she thought she was experiencing false labor. She went to bed.

At about 1:30 A.M. on the twelfth, she woke up. Her contractions were coming more often and getting more intense. "Maybe we should call the doctor now," she said. When she told the doctor her contractions were coming every twenty minutes, the doctor told her to come to the hospital right away.

Didi and I had made arrangements for one of our nephews, who lived nearby, to watch A.J. when Didi went into labor. By the time he got to our apartment, at about 2:00 A.M., Didi's contractions were coming less than ten minutes apart.

The cab ride from our apartment to the hospital takes about twenty minutes. When we arrived, the admitting nurse sent Didi to be seen right away. Didi had wanted to have an epidural, which she had done with A.J., but the doctor who examined her said it was too late. She was already seven centimeters dilated. When she said she felt like she needed to use the bathroom, the doctor advised against it. That sensation, she said, was the baby being born. They took us straight to a delivery room, and less than an hour later, Didi gave birth.

Oscar Eugene Gluck was born on February 12, 2008, at

3:37 A.M., weighing six pounds, five ounces. (Oscar gets his first and middle names from one of Didi's grandfathers and my father, respectively; A.J.'s middle name, Juliana, is a derivation of Julian, Didi's father's name.)

When A.J. was born, I literally had fallen to the ground. Didi, the doctor, and the nurses thought I had passed out; in fact I was overwhelmed with joy. My collapse was an involuntary form of celebration, like Björn Borg falling to his knees after winning Wimbledon. This time, at the appearance of Oscar, what I experienced was an involuntary shake of my head. "How," my body seemed to be asking, "did this happen?"

The birth of any child carries with it an air of incredulousness, but Oscar's arrival was more incredible than usual. Before long, my parents, my siblings, and Didi's mom came to meet him. Everyone seemed struck by a similar sense of awe.

A.J. was happy to have a little brother, but to be sure she didn't feel overlooked in the wake of his arrival, we got her a cat she named Mouse. (A.J. has always had a well-developed sense of irony.) Because Oscar is almost five years younger than A.J., people who don't know about my illness sometimes wonder if he was an "accident." A.J. teases him about that sometimes. She also calls Mouse her "consolation prize."

The fact is, having Oscar was probably the most intentional thing Didi and I have ever done. He couldn't have been more wanted.

3.

MAYBE IT WAS Oscar's birth. Or maybe it was because I was headed into deeper water, medically speaking. In either case,

I decided to see Dr. Paul Richardson, a renowned myeloma expert at the Dana-Farber Cancer Institute in Boston. By chance, my parents had had dinner one night with friends whose daughter had been treated by Dr. Richardson, and they had recommended him highly. Before my disease had advanced, I hadn't felt the need to reach out to him. Now I did.

Originally from Great Britain, Dr. Richardson has a cheerful manner, a twinkle in his eye, and a fundamentally optimistic outlook. He and his colleagues at Dana-Farber have spearheaded the development of many of the new myeloma therapies that have transformed the way the disease is treated and dramatically extended its survival rates.

At our first appointment, Dr. Richardson characterized my disease as Stage 1 multiple myeloma—it was official now, but at least I was in the lowest risk staging category—and laid out his vision for treatment. He told me I would likely need chemotherapy and a stem cell transplant at some point, but for now he recommended careful monitoring and monthly infusions of Zometa. He was aware of the jawbone issues associated with that drug, but based on the most recent studies available, which showed that the drug could not only help prevent bone damage in myeloma patients but could also extend their lives, he believed that the benefits outweighed the risks.

Because I was still relatively young, he said, his goal was to deploy the various available myeloma therapies as slowly as possible—"Keep your powder dry" was his exact phrase—to keep me alive and well for as long as possible. As Dr. Gruenstein had done, he made a point of mentioning that a number of promising myeloma treatments were in the pipeline and more were being developed. He also made a point of noting I was young, otherwise healthy, and had no family history of myeloma or other cancers. "That's good news," he said.

Other than a cure, the most valuable coin in the cancer realm is hope. Hope is like medicine for the spirit. What radiation and chemotherapy do for the body, hope does for the soul. I immediately liked him.

My brother, Andy, who lives outside Boston, went with me to that appointment, and such visits went on to become a regular ritual. Ostensibly, Andy accompanied me for emotional support and to be a second set of ears. But over time, the visits also became improbably enjoyable social occasions. You might think that physicians' waiting rooms and hospital cafeterias would not be great places to sit and talk, but the truth is, they gave us a rare opportunity to catch up without kids, wives, or others to interrupt us. If it was a little unusual, it was also delightful.

I had told Dr. Gruenstein that I planned to see Dr. Richardson, and he couldn't have been more understanding. As a myeloma specialist, Dr. Richardson had probably forgotten more about the disease than Dr. Gruenstein, who treated a variety of cancers, would ever know, he said. The three of us agreed on an arrangement in which Dr. Richardson would direct my care from Boston and Dr. Gruenstein would administer it in New York.

In the course of taking me on as a patient, Dr. Richardson had ordered another round of the usual myeloma tests. Although I still had no new lesions, my M protein levels were inching up.

Another challenge of learning to live with a long-term incurable illness is learning how to live with active disease while not doing anything about it, sometimes for months or years at a time. Medically speaking, strategies such as "keeping your powder dry" and "watchful waiting" make perfect sense. But as a patient—a real-life, actual human being with a disease simmering inside you that unapologetically intends to kill you—you want to fight back. In the face of such a serious problem, inaction feels deeply, maddeningly unsatisfying. You want to get any trace of disease out of you or at least tamp it down to undetectable levels *now*. You nod in agreement when the doctors tell you to sit tight, but what you really want to do is scream, "*Do something!*"

4.

ON FEBRUARY 1, 2009, the Pittsburgh Steelers were set to face the Arizona Cardinals in Tampa, Florida, in Super Bowl XLIII. My college friend Jeff, an actor who was doing voice-over work for the NFL as a side gig, was able to get us and our friends Randy and Eric tickets. The four of us had done similar trips before, but not since I had gotten sick.

I have unusual sports allegiances. Despite living in New York, I'm a Boston Red Sox and Pittsburgh Steelers fan. I follow those teams because when we were kids, my brother, who is two years older than I am, was a New York Yankees and Dallas Cowboys fan. As a good younger sibling does, I backed his teams' archenemies. I was particularly obsessed with the Steelers. I knew everything there was to know about each year's team (complete roster, full schedule, and so on), wore a Steelers varsity jacket with JON embroidered on it practically every day in grade school, and once badgered my parents into taking me to Pittsburgh to see the team play in their home stadium. The opportunity to see the Steelers play in the Super Bowl was a childhood wish come true. We flew to Tampa on Friday night, went to invitation-only parties on Friday and Saturday, thanks to Jeff's NFL connection, then attended the game on Sunday evening.

To some degree, trips with old friends are inevitably about turning back the clock, and I couldn't have been happier about that. For seventy-two hours, for the first time in as long as I could remember, no one talked about cancer, and I didn't think about it. That felt great, as did the Steelers' 27–23 victory, pulled out on a spectacular touchdown pass in the final seconds of the game.

If there's one thing I love about sports, it's the possibility of miraculous outcomes.

5.

WHEN I WAS a kid, my father would play catch in the backyard with me and my brother and shoot baskets with us in our driveway, often until well after dark and sometimes, in the dead of winter, until our hands were so raw we could still feel the sting in our fingertips the next morning. As I got older, he, my mother, my brother, and I played golf together (my sisters weren't interested), and we all skied together as a family. As it is for many fathers and their children, playing sports wasn't just something fun for us to do; it was a common language and a way to bond, a portal for our connection.

Golf was a particular passion for my father. He approached the game not with a country club attitude but in a populist, Arnold Palmer kind of way. (He and Palmer were born in the same year, and my father idolized him.) My father was a self-taught player who hadn't taken up the sport until his mid-thirties and had then studied and practiced his way to becoming a single-digit handicapper.

He started teaching me the game when I was eight or nine. He patiently tolerated my childhood fits of rage at the driving range when I would fail to keep my left arm straight or hit down and through the ball or execute whatever other invariably helpful instruction he was offering, and suffered through years of me hacking my way around fairways as a beginner. I honest-to-God shot a 149 once, and somehow it didn't bother him.

Eventually, I learned how to make my way through a round in a less humiliating fashion, and our outings became a regular source of joy. In high school and college, when I was home for the summer, he, one of his friends or my mother, and my brother and I would play almost every weekend, sometimes on both Saturday and Sunday, occasionally two rounds in a day. It wasn't just the game I found compelling; it was everything the game involved: my father and I putting on our spikes together in the locker room and getting coffee in Styrofoam cups at the screen-doored snack shop; the occasional three-hundred-yard drive, crisply struck 9-iron, or long, snaking putt that found the hole; the high-fives and fist bumps, the groans and the swearing; reliving shots over a beer or a Coke at the nineteenth hole. As a child, even as a teenager, even in my twenties, I had a sense of being allowed into a secret world, my father's world. He never made a thing of it; he just included me. The message he sent was that he enjoyed having me around. Is there a more valuable gift a parent can give a child?

After college, I moved around the country for various jobs, but my father and I still played golf when we could. On one memorable round I played with him and three of his friends, I somehow managed to shoot a 79, the first and only time I ever broke 80. I'm not sure who was happier, him or me. Actually, I am sure. My father was.

You might not think that golf would be a casualty of my illness, but it was. As a right-handed player, the weight shift involved puts too much pressure on my left hip. Fly-fishing, however, was another story. My father was well aware of my obsession with angling and enjoyed hearing stories of my travels and seeing pictures of the fish I caught. My mother told me he liked to show them to his friends. But he had never cast a fly line.

On Sunday, June 21, 2009, a month short of his eightieth birthday, I took my father fly-fishing for the first time. It was Father's Day. When I had realized he was turning eighty, I'd decided that the time was now. Although he was in good health, eighty is eighty, and although I had no active symptoms, cancer is cancer. Just as my diagnosis had driven me to spend as much time as I could with my kids, it led me to enjoy my parents' company as much as possible. As far as the Father's Day idea goes, sometimes the obvious choice is the best one.

When presented with an opportunity to try something new, my father often responded with something like "That sounds great. Let me think about it." It's not that he wasn't open to new experiences. He was just deliberate. When I asked him if he'd like to go fishing with me, he paused for a moment; then he said, "Yes."

My father had had a successful career. When I was growing up, he worked for my mother's father in a family printing business, then teamed with a partner to launch a magazine called *Wilderness Camping* that was eventually sold to the publishing giant Ziff-Davis (my father liked to tell the story of a last-minute boardroom bluff that sealed the deal that might have even been true). Although my father was on the marketing, not editorial, side of that operation, his involvement in it helped spark my interest in journalism. My father also served as the president of the board of education in our hometown and helped spearhead the construction of a much-needed new high school, one of his proudest achievements. When our family moved to Massachusetts when I was a teenager, my father took a job with a company called New England Business Services, then started his own direct marketing consulting firm, which he ran until the early 2000s, when he retired.

Despite all that, nothing ever meant more to him than his family. In addition to my siblings and me, he and my mother have nine grandchildren and six great-grandchildren. I know he's not unique in the history of parents and grandparents in this respect, but it always felt as though there was never anything my father wouldn't do for us. He came to our plays and our ball games. He attended our graduations. He called frequently just to say hello or to share a joke. When I got sick, he knew how to check in without being obtrusive, a rare gift.

On the weekend my father and I decided to go fishing together, my parents rendezvoused with Didi, A.J., Oscar, and me at my mother-in-law's in Amherst. It was a convenient meeting point, and I knew of a nearby river, the Swift, that was just right for first-time anglers.

My father and I headed out at 7:30 A.M. Because it is the law in Massachusetts, we stopped for breakfast at a Dunkin' Donuts, then drove to the river access point, where I had arranged for us to meet a guide.

A good fishing guide is invaluable. They know where the fish tend to be and which flies are most effective on a given river at a given time. I also hired a guide so I wouldn't have to teach my father how to fish. I thought it might make him uncomfortable. That way, I could outsource the instructional part of the day, then fish with him after that. My father was also a good listener and an eager student, a "coachable athlete," as the expression goes. I knew he'd be open to a professional's advice.

In the parking lot, we met our guide, a brash, plainspoken redhead named Marla, who I later learned is something of a

legend in western Massachusetts guide circles. After exchanging hellos, rigging our rods, and sliding into our waders, we set off.

The path from the lot to the river runs through a stand of
pine trees that smells like Christmas and is carpeted with old
pine needles. It is mostly smooth, but there are some roots. A
few steps along the way, my father stumbled. His rod went
flying, his sunglasses sailed off his head, and he lay on the
ground in a pile. Luckily, he was fine. We had narrowly
averted violating the first rule of the Sentimental Father's
Day Father-Son Outing: Don't kill the father.

The Swift River has a pretty, tucked-away quality to it.
Tree-lined banks hold cool, fern green water. Although Massachusetts Route 9 is nearby, you feel as if you are in a se-
cluded forest. A sense of peacefulness abides. Marla led my
father to an open spot where she could teach him to cast, and
I walked downstream twenty yards or so to find a patch of
water to fish myself.

The fly cast is, in a sense, an upside-down golf swing. In
both instances, you have to generate maximum acceleration
of the equipment in question (the golf club or fly rod) at
precisely the right moment (when a golfer strikes the ball or
when an angler stops the rod on the fore cast to "shoot" the
fly line forward) to achieve the intended result.

Naturally, I was stealing looks upstream to check out how
my father's casting was going. When I saw he was getting the
hang of it, I felt an unexpected sense of pride. It brought to
mind a scene from *A River Runs Through It* in which the
preacher father stands on the bank of a Montana river and
beams with satisfaction at the sight of his young sons fishing. If it hadn't been clear to me before that my father and I
were engaged in some kind of role reversal, it was definitely
apparent now.

Maybe half an hour later, Marla signaled to me to join her and my father. They were ready to fish. We took a few steps toward the far bank, spread out enough to each have our own runs, and had at it. Before long, I heard "Set!"—the guide command that translates to "Lift your rod, dumbass! A fish just ate your fly." My father did as instructed, and sure enough, his line went tight. He had a fish on. While Marla talked him through the process of netting his catch, I walked over to see what he'd landed.

My father's first ever fish caught on a fly was a gorgeous eleven-inch rainbow trout, its namesake pattern lit up in its full prismatic palette by the New England summer sun. As much as anything, my father seemed stunned. *Did that really just happen? Can a fish honestly be that beautiful? Can catching one truly make a man this happy?*

Over the next few hours, my father and I caught more rainbows and some equally pretty brook trout, each of us enjoying the other's successes as much as, if not more than, our own. We didn't catch anything all that big or rack up impressive numbers, but that was fine. No one was keeping score.

By around 12:30, things were slowing down, and the time we'd booked with Marla was coming to an end. She moved us to a new spot. At first, not much happened. But then I got a fish on the line, and a moment later, I heard "Set!" My father and I were both hooked up at the same time, a relative rarity.

In his years of playing golf, my father had notched three holes in one. Although "doubling up" in fishing isn't anywhere near as unusual, you wouldn't have known it from the smile on his face.

That afternoon, we had lunch back at my mother-in-law's. My father normally drove whenever my parents traveled, but when I walked them to the car afterward, it was my mother who got behind the wheel. She told me later that he had slept the whole way home.

<h1 style="text-align:center">6.</h1>

IN MARCH 2010, my high school friend Rich died of an aggressive form of colon cancer. He was forty-four. He had a wife and two young children. Later that spring, a memorial service was held for him at our school. Rich had had a 50,000-watt smile that reflected his equally bright spirit. Everyone who eulogized him talked about that smile. That evening, a group of us parked our cars around the school's football field. We played some of Rich's favorite music—Crosby, Stills, Nash & Young, Van Morrison—and swapped stories about him. It was a sad night.

Since I was diagnosed with cancer, I have lost a number of friends, family members, and coworkers to the disease. In addition to Rich, a former *New York* magazine colleague, John Homans, died of colon cancer. He was sixty-two. My father's sister, my aunt Rena, had lung cancer, and my uncle Milton, Rena's twin, had liver cancer. The two of them died, incredibly enough, on the same day, at age eighty-nine.

Milton's daughter, my cousin Julie, was born with congenital heart problems and died when she was nine. I have childhood memories of her playing the violin in her family's living room on Long Island and of my parents leaving us with a babysitter to attend her funeral. Hanging on the same wall of our apartment as our other fishing photographs is a picture of Didi's father smiling proudly next to a trophy marlin. I am older now than he was when he passed away.

The longer you live with a serious illness, the more you

realize how lucky you are. You also ask yourself: *Why am I here? Why aren't they?*

7.

IN THE WINTER of 2009 and the spring of 2010, my disease progressed. Every scan and blood draw seemed to reveal a new issue, but for a time Dr. Richardson didn't want me to undergo further treatment. *Keep your powder dry.*

In April 2010, a PET scan showed that I had numerous lesions, from my skull to my neck to my spine. My scans were starting to look like the Swiss cheese images I had come across on the internet after I was first diagnosed. Of particular concern were two lesions on vertebrae in my neck and midback that had grown large enough to cause potentially serious problems, including paralysis.

Those lesions were also painful. Whenever I turned my head or twisted my body, they announced themselves in no uncertain terms. It's difficult enough to sit tight and keep your powder dry when your disease is not actively bothering you, but when you have overt symptoms, you not only want to beat back the underlying cause of your illness as fast as you can, you also want to treat its manifestations. If pain is your body's way of getting your attention, it works.

Pain also makes it hard to think about anything other than your disease. Try as you might to keep your illness in a box, that's difficult to do when you're in pain. Pain is a great decompartmentalizer. Pain will not be ignored.

Dr. Richardson ordered another round of radiation to be done as soon as possible. It was time to use some powder.

Because the new hot spots were in delicate locations, I decided to return to Dr. Dalton at Mount Sinai to treat them.

I was inclined to go back to him anyway. As it happened, a *New York Times* story at around that time had called attention to a radiation overdose at St. Vincent's that had left the victim "deaf, struggling to see, unable to swallow, burned, with his teeth falling out, with ulcers in his mouth and throat, nauseated, in severe pain and finally unable to breathe."

Radiation round three featured two new twists. Whereas the mapping tattoos for rounds one and two had been located on my hips and torso, respectively, where they were out of sight, one of the markings for round three was etched on my Adam's apple, where it was visible. That meant I might have to explain what that marking was to anyone who noticed it, including my children. Again Didi and I discussed telling A.J. and Oscar I had cancer, and again we decided they were too young. If they asked about the tattoo, I would tell them it was a weird freckle. Fortunately, they never asked.

Because the radiation needed to be especially precise to hit the vertebrae in question without damaging my heart and lungs, a special setup was required. A mesh face covering, not unlike a fencing mask, was custom fabricated to fit me. For each of my treatments, I would lie on my back, and the technicians would bolt the mask to a wooden board placed under my head and neck to keep me as still as possible. It was uncomfortable and claustrophobic, and it didn't make me feel any better that it made me look like Hannibal Lecter.

Over the next three and a half weeks, I had eighteen Lecter Mask sessions. Once again, the therapy eliminated the targeted lesions and alleviated my symptoms but did not induce a full remission.

I had been treated for cancer three times, but only one of the three treatments had really worked. I was starting to think of cancer as the Jason Voorhees character from the

Friday the 13th movies: a form of evil incarnate that, no matter what weapons you throw at it, will not die.

8.

ON MARCH 16, 2011, Geraldine Ferraro, the former congresswoman and first female vice presidential nominee to represent a major American political party, died. I not only felt for
her and her family, but I was shaken.

Congresswoman Ferraro was the first well-known person
with multiple myeloma I had become aware of after my diagnosis, and she had become something of a talisman for
me. The longer she lived, I reasoned, the longer I might live.
When I heard of her passing, a chill went through me. It was
not an auspicious sign.

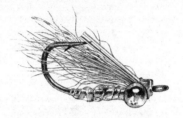

FOR THE FIRST eight years of my illness, my doctors had been playing Whac-a-Mole with my myeloma lesions, beating them back one by one with radiation. But my disease had become too widespread for that. Dr. Richardson decided it was time for me to start systemic therapy.

The history of cancer and cancer treatment dates back millennia. In 2016, in a cave in South Africa, researchers found what they identified as evidence of bone cancer, a cauliflower-like tumor on the foot of an early hominid who lived 1.7 million years ago. Some five thousand years ago, an ancient Egyptian papyrus described the process by which breast tumors were removed by cauterization. The papyrus also noted that there seemed to be no effective treatment for the disease. Spanish scientists studying a 4,600-year-old Egyptian skull found cut marks around lesions identified by previous researchers as metastasized brain cancer; the shape of the cuts indicated that they had been made by a metal tool.

Some 2,400 years ago, Hippocrates used the words *karcinos* and *karcinoma,* terms that refer to crabs, to describe the scourge of cancer. A cancerous tumor and the tangle of swollen blood vessels around it, the ancient Greek physician believed, resembled the body and legs of a crab. The metaphor has since been used to evoke the hard shell of certain tumors and the pain the disease can cause, reminiscent of the sharp pinch of a crab's claws.

About 250 years after Hippocrates, another Greek physician, Galen, described tumors with the word *oncos* (Greek for "growth," "lump," or "burden"). Fast-forward another four centuries, and the Roman physician Celsus noted that even after surgical removal the disease returned. Yet surgeons understandably continued their efforts to cut out and cauterize tumors. In the 1700s, physicians such as the Scottish surgeon John Hunter offered guidelines on which cancers might be most appropriate to operate on (those that had not invaded surrounding tissue). With the development of anesthesia in the mid-1800s, surgeries grew more aggressive, with operations such as radical mastectomies becoming common. Radiation joined the treatment arsenal at the dawn of the twentieth century, with Wilhelm Conrad Röntgen's discoveries, and both surgery and radiation continue to undergo refinements to this day.

Chemotherapy, or the use of chemical toxins to kill cancerous cells, dates back to the 1940s. Widely referred to as "the father of chemotherapy," Dr. Sidney Farber, a pathologist turned cancer researcher who began his career at Children's Hospital in Boston and went on to found what is now the Dana-Farber Cancer Institute, where Dr. Richardson works, had been studying childhood leukemia. A type of blood cancer in which white blood cells grow uncontrollably, leukemia can lead to infections, abnormal bleeding, nutritional problems, and multiple organ failure. At the time Farber began his work, children diagnosed with the disease often died within weeks and rarely survived for more than several months. Because leukemia is an especially difficult form of cancer to treat, Farber reasoned that unlocking its mysteries could lead to a cure for other cancers as well.

Inspired by a fellow researcher who had successfully treated anemia, another blood disease, with folate, a B vitamin needed for the healthy functioning of blood cells, Farber theorized that folate might also be an effective way to treat children with leukemia. In the summer of 1946, he conducted an experiment in which he injected a number of his patients with folic acid, a manufactured form of folate. But the experiment backfired. Instead of deterring the growth of leukemia cells, the folate accelerated their growth, likely hastening the children's death, and the injections were quickly stopped. Despite its morally questionable methods and disastrous results (with more rigorous regulations in place today, such an experiment would likely not be allowed), the experiment gave Farber an idea: If folate sped the growth of leukemia cells, perhaps a drug with properties opposite those of folate could halt that growth.

In September 1947, he injected a patient with a synthetic "antifolate" he had obtained known as pteroylaspartic acid, or PAA, but the treatment was ineffective. Several months later, in December, however, he injected another patient with a modified version of PAA called aminopterin. This time, the results were striking. The patient's white cell count not only stopped rising but began falling, eventually returning to almost normal.

In June 1948, Farber published a paper in *The New England Journal of Medicine* documenting the fact that ten of the sixteen children he and his team had treated with aminopterin had responded to the therapy and five had lived for four to six months after their treatment, far longer than the average survival time in those years. Farber's antifolates weren't a cure, but they demonstrated a game-changing principle: Cancer cells could be killed with chemicals.

Another seminal moment in the history of chemotherapy came during World War II. On the night of December 2, 1943, German pilots bombed an important Allied port in Bari, Italy, sinking seventeen ships and killing more than a thousand American and British military personnel along with hundreds of civilians. The surprise attack was dubbed "Little Pearl Harbor." Among the ships sunk that night was the *John Harvey*, an American vessel that was secretly carrying mustard gas bombs.

The German attack released the gas into the air and water, sickening and eventually killing scores more people. Because the Allies had intended to use the poison gas only if Adolf Hitler engaged in chemical warfare but were afraid that the Germans might now use the news of an Allied shipment of mustard gas to justify such a tactic, the U.S. and British governments attempted to cover up the incident. In the meantime, in the course of investigating the disaster, a young chemical warfare specialist, Lieutenant Colonel Stewart Francis Alexander, determined that the additional casualties had been caused by the toxic effects of mustard gas. In particular, he noted the devastating effect the substance had on white blood cells.

Alexander documented his findings in a report called "Final Report of the Bari Mustard Casualties." Although the report was immediately classified, Alexander's superior officer in the Chemical Warfare Service, Colonel Cornelius P. "Dusty" Rhoads, was intrigued by his discoveries. As the head of New York's Memorial Hospital for the Treatment of Cancer and Allied Diseases in his civilian life, Rhoads was interested in mustard gas's cell-destroying characteristics and theorized that the agent, if employed in a carefully controlled way, might be used to kill cancer cells.

In 1945, based on Alexander's report and related work being done at Yale University showing that another form of mustard gas could kill tumors, Rhoads persuaded the philanthropists Alfred P. Sloan, Jr., and Charles F. Kettering to fund the Sloan Kettering Institute for cancer research (now Memorial Sloan Kettering Cancer Center, the hospital where I saw Dr. Boland) in New York. There, Rhoads and other scientists experimented with mustard gas derivatives.

In 1949, Mustargen (generic name mechlorethamine hydrochloride) was used to successfully treat a form of lymphoma, a type of blood cancer. It was the first chemotherapy drug approved by the Food and Drug Administration.

In the 1950s and 1960s, researchers began to explore how they might use a combination of chemotherapy drugs, rather than a single agent, to fight cancer. The rationale was that lower doses of several drugs might kill more cancer cells than a higher dose of a single drug, in part because the multiple-drug approach might kill a wider range of cancer cells with different abnormalities and vulnerabilities. Hitting cancer with an array of drugs in that way might also slow down the disease's ability to develop resistance to chemotherapy agents. The first combination-drug approach was used in the mid-1960s to treat Hodgkin's lymphoma. It was named MOPP after its components: mechlorethamine hydrochloride, Oncovin (also known as vincristine), procarbazine hydrochloride, and prednisone.

As effective as chemotherapy can be, it is also problematic. Even as it kills cancer cells, it kills healthy cells, often leading to severe, and in some cases fatal, side effects. As a result, researchers began looking to develop more targeted, less toxic therapies.

In the late 1990s, an improved understanding of the biology of cancer and the molecular mechanisms that cause tumors to grow led researchers to develop the fourth of the so-called five pillars of cancer treatment: so-called targeted therapy, or treatment that uses drugs to attack specific substances that cancer cells need to survive and spread (with less damage to healthy cells and fewer side effects than chemotherapy).

Targeted therapies work in numerous ways. They might

block signals that cause cancer cells to grow, starve cancer cells of hormones they need to survive, or deliver cell-killing substances to cancer cells. The two main types of targeted therapy are referred to as small-molecule medicines and monoclonal antibodies. Small-molecule medicines are so named because they are little enough to get inside cancer cells and kill them. Their generic names end in *ib*.

In 2001, a drug called Gleevec (generic name imatinib) became one of the first well-known targeted therapies. Developed by Dr. Brian Druker, an oncologist at Oregon Health & Science University, Gleevec has helped turn chronic myelogenous leukemia, or CML, from a deadly disease into a frequently treatable condition managed by a daily pill.

Monoclonal antibodies can't enter cells. Instead, they attack cells from the outside. Some do so directly, attaching themselves to cancer cells, then triggering a series of events inside those cells that cause them to self-destruct. Others "flag" cancer cells for destruction by alternate methods. Still, others deliver chemotherapy directly to cancer cells while avoiding damage to other cells. The generic names of monoclonal antibodies end in *mab*. Most small-molecule drugs are administered as tablets or capsules, while most monoclonal antibodies are given intravenously.

Targeted therapies have since been developed to treat everything from breast cancer and lung cancer to colorectal cancer and melanoma, and targeted therapy remains an area of intensive research, with dozens of new iterations in development.

Perhaps the form of cancer therapy that has received the most attention in recent years is the fifth and latest "pillar" of cancer care, immunotherapy. (Because certain drugs have multiple mechanisms of action by which they attack cancer, there is some overlap between the terms *targeted therapy* and *immunotherapy*.) Immunotherapy uses your body's own defenses to kill cancer, in essence turbocharging your immune system to attack malignant cells.

In the late nineteenth century, a Harvard-trained surgeon and cancer researcher named William B. Coley was the first modern-day doctor to explore the idea of immunotherapy (the idea of causing infection to cure disease dates back as far as 1550 B.C.). After observing that some cancer patients experienced tumor regression after developing an immune response to bacterial infections, Coley proceeded to develop a treatment that came to be known as Coley's toxins, a mixture of heat-killed bacteria he injected into patients in the hope of stimulating the body's "resisting powers." The therapy proved to be neither safe nor effective, but for his pioneering efforts in the field, Coley became known as "the father of cancer immunotherapy."

It wasn't until the 1970s and 1980s when researchers discovered the role so-called T cells (short for "thymus-derived cells") play in the human immune system, that researchers began to discover how to tap the body's own defenses to fight cancer. Today, immunotherapy takes several main forms.

Immune checkpoint inhibitors prevent cancer cells from evading detection and destruction by the immune system, a trick some cancer cells can perform.

Cancer vaccines are used to prevent certain cancers and treat others. Preventive vaccines work by decreasing the incidence of viruses, such as HPV, which can lead to cancers, such as cervical cancer. Therapeutic vaccines work in varying ways. A vaccine called Imlygic (generic name talimogene laherparepvec), for example, is used to treat advanced melanoma that can't be completely removed by surgery. It is made of a virus that has been genetically engineered to promote an immune response to cancer.

Adoptive cell transfer, also known as T-cell transfer therapy, is a technique in which a patient's own immune cells are collected, sent to a lab to be genetically modified, then infused back into the patient intravenously. The two main forms of adoptive cell transfer are known as tumor-infiltrating lymphocytes, or TILs, and CAR T-cell therapy.

Immunotherapy has proven to be remarkably successful in treating skin cancer, lung cancer, colorectal cancer, and certain blood cancers, including multiple myeloma, and is expected to be used to combat many more.

For decades, multiple myeloma was treated with a combination of radiation, chemotherapy (including a drug called melphalan, descended from the original class of chemotherapy drugs developed from mustard gas), and steroids such as prednisone, which by stopping white blood cells from traveling to areas where myeloma cells are causing damage can reduce the inflammation and pain the disease can cause. (Surgery is rarely used to treat myeloma; you can't cut out blood cells.) Those treatments had significant side effects and were only moderately effective, resulting in a five-year survival rate of just 25 percent.

In the 1990s, doctors began treating myeloma with a pair of new chemotherapy drugs called doxorubicin and vincristine, along with steroids. They also began using stem cell transplants to fight the disease. By the year 2000, the five-year survival rate for myeloma rose to 34 percent.

Today, the therapies available to treat multiple myeloma include radiation, chemotherapy, bone marrow and stem cell transplants, targeted therapies, and immunotherapy. With almost every passing year, outcomes have improved. In 2020, the five-year survival rate reached an all-time high of 61 percent.

2.

WHEN I SAW Dr. Richardson, a stem cell transplant, preceded by a round of high-dose chemotherapy, was (and still is by many doctors) considered the standard of care for myeloma patients in the phase of the disease I was in. No treatment has been proven to deliver better survival rates. But because a transplant is difficult and risky and can have damaging long-term effects, including causing secondary cancers; because I was young enough to be at risk for those complications; and because new targeted therapies and immunotherapies were showing unprecedented promise, Dr. Richardson chose to go a different route, at least as a next step. I could always have a transplant farther down the road.

The treatment Dr. Richardson prescribed was a protocol called RVD, an acronym for a trio of drugs that includes two targeted therapy drugs, Revlimid (generic name lenalidomide) and Velcade (generic name bortezomib), and a steroid called dexamethasone.

A so-called immunomodulatory agent, a medication used to either suppress or stimulate the body's immune system, Revlimid regulates the interactions between myeloma cells and the bone marrow in which they grow, reducing the growth of cancer cells.

The drug has a complex and tragic history that traces back to a medication called thalidomide. Introduced in 1953 as a tranquilizer and later marketed by its German manufacturer as a treatment for anxiety, insomnia, and morning sickness, thalidomide was removed from the European market in 1961 after it became clear that it could cause severe birth defects, including the absence of bones and the malformation or absence of arms and legs. Some ten thousand infants are estimated to have been affected by the drug. About 40 percent of them died around the time of birth.

Thalidomide was never given FDA approval in the United States, but it had been widely distributed through clinical testing. The resulting furor pushed Congress to amend, in 1962, the Federal Food, Drug, and Cosmetic Act of 1938 to require drug manufacturers to prove both the effectiveness and the safety of their products and disclose information about side effects. Thalidomide, in effect, inspired modern drug regulation.

Yet research continued on the drug. Because the time and money involved in drug development are so significant, researchers rarely abandon interesting drugs. Instead, they seek other uses for them.

Less than three years after thalidomide was withdrawn from the market, researchers discovered that the drug's anti-inflammatory effects could reduce a painful complication of leprosy called erythema nodosum leprosum, or ENL. As researchers continued to study the medication, it was found to be useful in certain palliative care situations and as a treatment for HIV-related conditions. And in the early 1990s, researchers discovered that thalidomide could be used to inhibit something called angiogenesis.

Angiogenesis is the mechanism by which new capillaries proliferate, a process critical not only to embryogenesis (the process by which a fertilized egg becomes an embryo) and wound healing but also to tumor progression. Cancers, it turns out, recruit the growth of neighboring blood vessels in order to expand and flourish.

Dr. Judah Folkman, a Harvard Medical School professor, was the pioneer who launched the field of angiogenesis research, and in 1971, he published an article in *The New England Journal of Medicine* in which he hypothesized that if solid-tumor cancers could be thwarted in their attempt to hijack capillary growth, the tumors would wither and disappear. Folkman later found that certain blood cancers were also dependent on angiogenesis for their survival.

In the late 1990s and early 2000s, researchers tested thalidomide's ability to suppress multiple myeloma, particularly in patients whose disease had recurred and was resisting treatment, so-called relapsed or refractory disease. A derivative of thalidomide called lenalidomide, marketed under the brand name Revlimid, was developed by the pharmaceutical giant Celgene as a more potent molecular analog of the drug and one that also has fewer side effects. In June 2006, less than three years after I learned I was sick, the FDA approved lenalidomide for the treatment of relapsed or refractory multiple myeloma.

There is another notable chapter in Revlimid's history. In 2017, Celgene agreed to pay $280 million to settle claims that it had marketed Revlimid and another thalidomide variant called Thalomid for unapproved uses. The crux of the legal case was that although Celgene had received FDA approval to sell the drugs as treatments for multiple myeloma, the company had inappropriately marketed it to treat other cancers.

The case is a telling example of the issues raised by so-called off-label drug use, in which a drug approved for a specific application is used as treatment for a disease or patient group in which it has not been rigorously tested for safety and efficacy.

Patients and doctors are often eager to use off-label applications of drugs, especially to treat diseases with no known effective therapies. In the absence of viable alternatives, they argue, the potential benefits outweigh the risks. Many effective therapies that have gone on to gain FDA approval have been discovered through off-label use, including treatments for AIDS and many cancers. The AIDS epidemic, in particular, brought the issues of off-label drug use and sped-up drug approvals to the forefront. The landmark Food and Drug Administration Modernization Act, passed in 1997, is a reflection of those efforts.

To balance the value of off-label drug use against safety and efficacy concerns, regulators have largely allowed the practice but with certain caveats. Generally speaking, the more evidence there is that a drug is safe and effective, the more latitude it's given for off-label use. The burden of responsibility is placed on physicians to make sure that their patients understand the risks of off-label use and consent to it.

In the Celgene suit, it was decided that the company had pushed too hard in encouraging doctors to prescribe Thalomid and Revlimid for cancers other than multiple myeloma. Nevertheless, because so many cancers remain incurable, the practice of off-label drug use in cancer care is likely to remain high. A 2021 article in the *International Journal of Environmental Research and Public Health,* titled "Off-Label Medication: From a Simple Concept to Complex Practical Aspects," cited literature surveys that had found that up to 50 percent of cancer therapy occurred in an off-label regimen.

In "The Evolving Role and Utility of Off-Label Drug Use in Multiple Myeloma," an article published in the journal *Exploration of Targeted Anti-tumor Therapy,* also in 2021, the authors noted that off-label drug use has played a pivotal role in the development of myeloma therapies. "The treatment landscape for multiple myeloma (MM) has dramatically changed over the last three decades," they wrote, "moving from no US Food and Drug Administration approvals and two active drug classes to over 19 drug approvals and at least eight different active classes." This history, they continued, "provides a striking example of how the common prescribing practice of off-label drug use is used within a single disease setting, how this practice impacts the introduction of novel therapies, results in varied clinical trial designs, and eventually modifies clinical practice."

Velcade, the second of the three RVD drugs, belongs to a class of targeted therapy medicines called proteasome inhibitors. Originally known as PS-341, it was developed through a collaboration between the National Cancer Institute and the pharmaceutical company ProScript. The drug was first studied as a treatment for AIDS and muscular dystrophy, but when scientists realized that that effort was going to take longer than expected, a ProScript chemist named Julian Adams suggested it be investigated as a way to fight cancer.

Since the mid-1990s, scientists had known that a group of protein chains called a proteasome was required for cell survival and growth. Present in all cells, proteasomes eliminate excess or damaged proteins. They have been likened to a biological garbage disposal.

If proteasomes were responsible for eliminating damaged or harmful proteins in the cell, Dr. Adams hypothesized, they might also be responsible for removing beneficial proteins, including proteins that help fight off cancer. If PS-341 could slow down the action of proteasomes, it might also slow down the destruction of those valuable cancer-fighting cells. His thinking gave rise to a whole new class of anticancer drugs called proteasome inhibitors.

To test PS-341 as a cancer-fighting agent, Dr. Adams reached out to the National Cancer Institute. After early experiments with mice found that PS-341 significantly reduced cell growth in a variety of cancers, the drug was tested for use in multiple myeloma. Along with Dr. Adams, one of the leaders of that effort was Dr. Kenneth Anderson, an NCI-supported researcher and the director of the multiple my-eloma program at the Dana-Farber Cancer Institute.

In 2000, in a phase I clinical trial, researchers were sur-prised to find that a myeloma patient given a very low dose of PS-341 to test for its safety went into complete remission. After further tests at Dana-Farber and other sites (Dr. Rich-ardson was one of the principal investigators, as he had been for the development of Revlimid), PS-341 was approved by the FDA in 2003 to treat multiple myeloma and was given the brand name Velcade.

The third of the three RVD drugs, dexamethasone, is one of the steroids used to reduce inflammation in people under-going cancer treatment.

In 2010, just a year before I began RVD myself, Dr. Rich-ardson and a group of his colleagues had published the results of a landmark study they conducted in which fully 100 percent of the sixty-six patients who had undergone RVD therapy alone for newly diagnosed and active myeloma showed at least a partial response or better, with a signifi-cant number experiencing deep or complete remissions, in some cases lasting for many years. The RVD protocol, which Dr. Richardson and others had begun developing in 2004, became a new standard of care, one that doesn't require a transplant. Given my age and relatively good health, Dr. Richardson told me he expected me to do well on the treat-ment.

3.

REVLIMID IS TAKEN in pill form. Velcade was given intrave-nously at the time (and can now be given by injection). Dexa-methasone is administered intravenously. In my case, I would take the Revlimid every day for three weeks out of every four and have the Velcade and "dex" administered weekly by IV at Dr. Gruenstein's office. That regimen would last for six months. After a round of pre-authorization hassles with my insurance company (by now I was on a first-name basis with Dr. Gruenstein's pre-auth coordinator, Tiffany), I was approved to start the medications.

Because Revlimid has potentially life-threatening side effects, special procedures are required to obtain the drug. Instead of acquiring it from a standard pharmacy, you get it from what's called a specialty pharmacy, and you're required to complete a telephone survey and discuss the potential side effects with a nurse practitioner every month. Only then are you mailed your prescription.

The long list of the problems RVD can cause—heart attack, stroke, deep vein thrombosis, birth defects, peripheral neuropathy—that you review each month would be funny if it weren't so frightening. The number of times a complete stranger asks you if you are "sexually active with a woman who still has her womb and may be or could become pregnant," then reminds you that you "must use a latex condom whenever engaging in sexual intercourse to prevent the possibility of birth defects," all of it clearly read from a script, often with the robotic indifference of a DMV clerk issuing driver's licenses, however, is comical.

To prevent and manage the side effects of the RVD, the so-called supportive medications I had to take included aspirin (to prevent a heart attack, stroke, or blood clots), Zofran (to relieve nausea), Bactrim (to guard against bacterial infections), Valtrex (to fend off viral infections such as herpes and shingles), Peridex (a prescription mouthwash that blocks mouth sores associated with RVD), and Prilosec. The Prilosec is used to impede ulcers caused by the aspirin. That was a first for me: a side effect medicine needed to treat a side effect medicine.

To manage my pharmacological routine, I bought one of those pill dispensers with S M T W T F S marked on it to indicate the days of the week and filled each compartment with the appropriate pills, a mix of capsules and tablets in an array of purple, blue, and white. To keep A.J. from getting suspicious—she was eight now and curious about just about everything—I hid the dispenser in my underwear drawer.

Although I was forty-six years old, taking all of those pills, from that sort of dispenser no less, made me feel like I was ninety. I started every day by popping a Prilosec and finished it by swishing my mouth with Peridex. Every day began and ended with cancer.

4.

THE DAY BEFORE I was scheduled to start my RVD treatment, my sisters came to my apartment to have brunch with me, Didi, A.J., and Oscar.

It was a Sunday. I picked up bagels and all the fixings from our local deli, and we sat around our dining room table to eat. I don't remember what we did after that, but if I had to guess, I'd say that Jen and Tina probably read or played games with A.J. and Oscar and we went to the park. The adults had become skilled in the art of acting normally in the face of abnormalcy.

When it was time to say goodbye, I walked Jen and Tina to the Union Square subway station. It was a strange place to say what I was about to say, but it was the only place I could say it. I didn't want A.J. and Oscar to overhear me. I thanked them for coming and for their love and support, both on that day and over the years. I told them I wasn't scared of starting the RVD therapy, which was a lie, and that I was actually eager to get on with it and start feeling better, which was true.

Then I asked them for a favor. In the event that I were to die from my treatment, I asked them if they would please help Didi look after A.J. and Oscar. Of course they would, they said. If the worst were to happen, I asked them if they would also try to help A.J. and Oscar see my death not as a tragedy but as an inevitable part of life. I asked them to encourage A.J. and Oscar to try to focus on the time we'd had together, not the time we didn't, and to remember that my spirit would always be a part of them. I encouraged them to look at things the same way. They promised they would do all of that.

Somehow the three of us got through my spiel with only a few tears. We hugged, said our goodbyes, and down the subway hole they went.

5.

ON MONDAY, MAY 2, 2011, Didi and I went to Dr. Gruenstein's office for my first RVD infusion. At the time, his treatment room was a small, simple space outfitted with five or six faux leather reclining chairs. You could think of them as Barca-Loungers, only for having your veins filled with toxic chemicals instead of watching football and eating chicken wings.

One of the nurses inserted my IV line for the Velcade and the dex and brought me a plastic cup that contained a blue-and-white pill, the Revlimid. She started the drip, and I downed the pill. She told me to let her know if I felt anything unusual once we got started, and I brushed her off. *Me? Ha! I sailed through three rounds of radiation therapy with*

*hardly any side effects! I have barely missed a day of work in
more than eight years since being diagnosed with cancer!
There is no way—*

Then I started to feel flushed, and red patches began to
appear on my arms, legs, and face. I was having an allergic
reaction to the RVD. I panicked. That was the best-known
therapy at that point for my disease. If I couldn't tolerate it,
then what? But a dose of IV Benadryl controlled the reaction, and I was able to proceed an hour or so later.

You know you're in the upside-down world of cancer
when the idea of proceeding with six months of difficult and
potentially fatal medical treatment makes you happy.

6 .

ON MONDAY, MAY 9, a week after I started my RVD treatment,
I had my second infusion. That night, the National Magazine Awards were held.

It was a heady time to work at *New York*. Adam Moss
had succeeded in restoring the magazine to its prior level of
excellence, winning multiple National Magazine Awards
and other honors along the way. That night, *New York* took
home the prizes for General Excellence and Best Magazine
Section. Because I oversaw the section in question, Adam
gave me, along with the others involved, a shout-out when he
accepted the award.

At the same time, my feelings about working at *New York*
had begun to change. It was beginning to dawn on me that
the kind of stress involved in producing a weekly magazine
with a daily website maybe wasn't the best thing for a cancer
patient. The RVD therapy was a much bigger deal than the
radiation treatments; it made my illness feel more real and
more taxing. A.J. was eight and Oscar was three, ages where

I enjoyed spending more and more time with them. My priorities were shifting. I still loved what I did; I just wanted to do a little less of it and maybe put it into better balance with the rest of my life.

After the National Magazine Awards ceremony, a group of us went to a restaurant in the West Village that had become something of a clubhouse for the magazine. Afterward, as I was walking home among the redbrick brownstones and cobblestone streets, I had the same feeling of surprised satisfaction I'd had in Washington Square Park the night I shipped the first issue of the magazine for lawyers and law students I had helped start. This time, however, I also felt a kind of emotional whiplash. One of my proudest professional achievements happened in the middle of one of the worst times in my personal life.

Cancer, of course, didn't care. Cancer is indifferent to timing.

7.

THAT SAME WEEK, Didi and I had plans to go to dinner for a friend's birthday. The restaurant where we were meeting, in Manhattan's East Village, was located across the street from a small city park. Our reservation was at eight, but because I was feeling tired from my treatment, I decided to leave work early and head to the park to rest for a few minutes.

By the time I got there, the sun was setting and just about all the park-goers were heading home. *Excellent*, I thought. *It will be nice and quiet.* I found an empty bench and lay down. Before long, a pair of teenagers walked up to the bench and stood over me. One of them said, "Excuse me, sir," then asked if he could use my cellphone. He said he had lost his and needed to call his mother to let her know when he would be home. By that time, I had lived in New York for more than fifteen years. I told him I wouldn't give him my phone, but I'd be happy to call his mother if he gave me her number. Then he lifted his T-shirt to reveal a revolver tucked into the waistband of his sweatpants. "Give me your phone, the watch, and the wallet," he said.

"Jesus," I blurted out. "I'm a cancer patient. I'm in the middle of having chemotherapy."

"Damn," he said. "I'm sorry."

For a moment, I thought I had run into an empathic mugger. Then he repeated his demand for my wallet, watch, and phone.

Somewhere I had heard that most thieves don't want your ID and credit cards—they just throw them away, anyway, to get rid of the evidence. They only want your money and anything they can sell. I handed over my phone, my watch, and the cash I was carrying—about $150—but asked if I could keep my wallet. (The only thing worse than getting mugged is having to go to the DMV to get a driver's license.)

They said I could keep the wallet. Then the kid who had been talking said, "Stay here for ten minutes and don't move. We'll be watching. If you move, we'll kill you."

I waited five minutes, then walked across the street to the restaurant. Didi and the two couples we were meeting were already seated. I told them what had happened and, despite the fact that I'd been instructed not to drink while I was undergoing RVD, ordered a double bourbon. My need to calm my nerves outweighed any worries I had about adverse drug reactions.

The truth is that the kids—and they were kids—who had robbed me had seemed as nervous as I was; I had never thought they would hurt me. I had the sense that it was their first holdup. I wasn't sure that the gun was even real—maybe it was a toy—or, if it was real, if it was loaded.

Didi and our friends asked if I wanted to call the police or just go home, but I told them I felt fine. I said I'd rather just forget about it and go ahead with our dinner.

Believe it or not, we had a nice evening. We ate and drank and talked about our kids, jobs, and lives and all the other usual subjects. Arguably the most unpleasant part of the night for me was the fact that the restaurant had a bone marrow item on the menu. I have no culinary objection to the dish; I used to enjoy it. But for reasons you might imagine, I'm no longer a fan.

By the next morning, all the fear and anxiety I had experienced the night before had alchemized into anger, and my mind buzzed with thoughts of revenge. I replayed the incident in my head, only this time I fought back. I had visions of returning to the park to look for my assailants.

On my way to work, I saw a police officer on the subway platform. I told him about the night before and asked what he thought might have happened if I had tried to fight back. I also asked if he thought the gun was real or loaded and if I should have reported the incident. He said that the gun had probably been real but not loaded. That way, if the kids got arrested, they would face a lesser charge.

So I should have fought back? That probably wouldn't have been a good idea, he said. The two teenagers were likely working with more experienced partners who were watching from nearby and might have jumped in; their guns would likely have been real and loaded. As for reporting the incident, he said, I could do that, but the odds of anyone getting arrested were low. The NYPD simply had more serious cases to worry about.

That night, Didi and I talked about the incident again. I told her I wondered if the teens had sensed that I was weak from my cancer treatment. "Like, I was the wounded giraffe, and they were lions on the veld."

8.

THE SIX MONTHS of RVD were a mixed bag. The pain from my bone lesions disappeared, and the treatments themselves didn't make me feel particularly sick. I was sometimes a little nauseous and tired afterward, but not too bad. Because RVD is an immunomodulatory therapy, not chemotherapy, I still didn't lose my hair. Still, there was damage.

Revlimid can cause severe dehydration, and I passed out several times because of it. Once I was at a Patti Smith concert with Didi. As I had done after I'd been mugged, I decided to take a chance on having a drink. Didi and I each had a beer and I also had a tequila shot. We were standing on the floor not far from the stage at a small venue, swaying along to a song, and *boom,* down I went. After I drank a few glasses of water and got some fresh air on the sidewalk, I felt better. We went back to the concert.

Another time I was playing miniature golf with A.J., Oscar, and Didi on a Saturday afternoon. There was no alcohol involved, but I had gone for a long walk that morning and hadn't had much water afterward. The next thing I knew, a stranger was gently shaking me and asking me if I was okay. Fortunately, Didi and the kids were a few holes ahead and didn't see anything, but the incident worried me. I didn't want to be forced to tell A.J. and Oscar that I had cancer; I wanted to tell them on my own terms. I'd gotten lucky that time, but what if that weren't the case next time?

That night, I told Didi what I was thinking. At her age,

A.J. was arguably old enough to understand, but Oscar was still in preschool, and we didn't want to tell one of them without telling both of them. It didn't seem fair to Oscar to keep him in the dark if we told his sister, and it didn't seem right to ask A.J. to keep a secret from her brother. We decided once again to keep the information to ourselves.

In what is obviously some kind of cosmic joke, Revlimid can cause both diarrhea and constipation. For me, the former led to more than one episode of desperate sprints to the bathroom. One day I was walking home from work when I suddenly had an urgent need to use the bathroom. Because it was early in my treatment, before I understood how serious the problem was, I decided to keep going instead of stopping somewhere to find a toilet. That was a mistake. Less than a block from my apartment, I was no longer able to control my bowels. I skulked past my doorman and took the stairs, not the elevator, upstairs. Fortunately, no one in my family was home. I showered, then rinsed out my jeans and underwear, put them into a garbage bag, and threw the whole mess down the garbage chute. Few things I've experienced because of my illness have been more upsetting or humiliating.

To address the issue, Dr. Richardson added yet another medication to my pharmacological lineup, a pill called cholestyramine. Revlimid can cause an immune-based reaction to an overproduction of bile in the gut; that's what leads to the diarrhea. Cholestyramine, which is commonly used to control cholesterol, also removes bile from your system and can minimize this effect.

The constipation, for its part, led to something called an anal fistula, an abnormal "tunnel" that forms between the anal canal in the colon and the skin of the buttocks that can be caused by excessive straining when you're trying to defecate. It required surgery to repair. After I got home from the operation, I noticed a small cut on my left earlobe. When I asked a surgeon friend how he thought I had wound up with a cut nowhere near the site of my procedure, he guessed that the doctor or a nurse had probably dropped a scalpel. "It happens," he said. "Things slip."

Revlimid can also cause severe muscle cramps, and I had those, too. Dr. Richardson had warned me to be careful: He had told me about an RVD patient of his who had suffered a leg cramp so sudden and painful that he fell and cracked two ribs. Even when I wasn't experiencing cramps, my muscles, especially the large ones, such as my quadriceps, felt hard, stiff, and painful, as though they were made of cement. Dr. Richardson recommended massages. They helped, but because they were painful, and expensive, I didn't do them that often. Stretching was a small help, but not much.

That was the fallout from the Revlimid. The Velcade caused me to lose the feeling in the tips of several fingers, and the dex brought with it the sleeplessness, restlessness, and anxiety that many steroids do. On the nights after each weekly treatment, I would sleep maybe two or three hours. I would babble at Didi and the kids to the point where they would have to gently ask me to lower my voice and calm down. If I exerted myself or got nervous, my heart would pound as though I had just done a set of wind sprints. On several occasions, the dex gave me heartburn so intense that I woke up in the middle of the night thinking I was having a heart attack. Because it can interfere with the functioning of the diaphragm, dex can also cause severe cases of hiccups. I've had episodes of six and seven hours. It's funny for about the first twenty minutes.

During my RVD treatment, I began having a recurring nightmare. I'm traveling, either from New York to somewhere else or from somewhere else to New York. The details vary—eating dinner in Rome, fishing in Oregon, taking in a blues show in Mississippi—but the gist of the dream is always the same: Something goes wrong—my flight is canceled; my hotel door is locked, and I can't get out; my cellphone isn't working, and I can't call an Uber—and no matter how hard I try, I can't get to where I want to go. In other words, there's a problem I desperately want to fix but can't because it's beyond my control. I feel frustrated and helpless.

That's another way my unconscious seems to express itself.

9.

THAT AUGUST, DIDI, A.J., Oscar, and I went to Wyoming for our usual family vacation. While we were there, I decided to take A.J. and Oscar fishing for the first time. The RVD had made me more conscious than ever of doing as much as I could with them while I was alive and well, and taking them fishing was high on my to-do list. I drove them to a small stream suited to beginners, showed them the basics of how to cast, and let A.J. have at it.

A handful of fish were rising within her range, and within five minutes, she hooked and landed a small, pretty cutthroat. I unhooked him, kissed him to thank him for his cooperation, and released him. Oscar was too young to cast by himself, but I hooked a fish for him, then handed him the rod and let him reel in his catch.

After each kid had caught and released a few more fish, we decided to call it a day. It was hot and sunny, and I didn't want the kids to get cranky. I wanted their first fishing outing to be a positive one. I figured I should quit while they were still smiling.

Back in the parking lot, I opened the tailgate of the SUV we had rented and broke out a cooler I had packed. The three of us ate peanut-butter-and-jelly sandwiches and cheddar cheese Goldfish and drank apple juice from plastic juice boxes. I have been lucky enough to dine at some pretty good restaurants, but nothing I have ever eaten tasted as good.

I have three snapshots from that day framed as a triptych that hangs on our apartment wall. One is of the first fish A.J. caught, another is a still life of the fly we used, and the third is of the three of us standing by the car. A.J. and I are holding our rods. Oscar has his hand in the bag of Goldfish. Everyone looks completely content.

10.

AFTER MY FINAL RVD infusion, a nurse removed my IV, bandaged my arm, and wished me good luck. (How many cancer-cursed souls have oncology nurses sent off with that wish?) She walked me to Dr. Gruenstein's office for a previously scheduled check-in, where he told me he was glad I was done and that things had gone relatively smoothly. Then he informed me that I would need to remain on Revlimid indefinitely, as maintenance therapy. That was the standard protocol, but somehow he had forgotten to communicate that to me. Or maybe he didn't want to put too much onto my plate at once.

Either way, it was an unwelcome surprise. One of the things that helps you get through cancer treatment is the idea that there's an end to it, that if you put your head down and bang it out, there will come a day, eventually, when it will be over. When you're done, you want to be *done* done.

Instead, I was confronted for the first time with a treatment that would never end. I put on a brave face (don't we all want to please our doctors?), but inside I was shaken. I took some solace in the fact that Revlimid is taken in pill form, meaning that I would no longer need weekly IV infusions, and that I would at least be off the Velcade and dex. I understood that staying on Revlimid could help keep me alive, and I was grateful for that. Still, was it too much to ask not to be on it forever?

11.

AFTER RVD, DOCTORS wait a month or two before retesting you to see if the treatment worked. It takes time for the therapy to achieve its full effect. Once again, I ran the gauntlet of tests: blood work, a PET scan, a marrow biopsy. Once again, I waited anxiously for the results.

Dr. Gruenstein called me early on a Tuesday morning. All my tests were negative. The RVD had worked spectacularly. The two greatest acronyms in cancer care are NED and CR: no evidence of disease and complete remission. That was my status.

Despite the fact that I was disease free for the first time in seven years, I didn't run around my office like a madman, and no cheery Jimmy Cliff songs popped into my head. It's not that I wasn't thrilled. I was. But I was also starting to learn that it was best to stay off the emotional roller coaster of highs and lows. It's too draining with a long-term illness. With every high, you set yourself up for a fall. With every low, you intensify the depth of your misfortune. It's better to seek a middle ground.

There's also a hard reality that tends to keep unbridled enthusiasm in check. When you know that your disease is bound to return, any success, no matter how welcome, comes with an asterisk. The wall of denial I had built after my first remission no longer served any purpose. This time, I was perfectly aware I was back on the clock.

12.

LIKE MANY OTHER magazines in the mid-2010s, *New York* was under intense economic pressure, as the internet continued to eat into its advertising revenue and drain its readership. It was becoming clear to me that layoffs were inevitable and that as a senior, relatively high-salaried employee, I was likely to lose my job. No matter how much I enjoyed working there, the risk of losing my income and medical insurance was too great for me to stay. One of the things cancer teaches you is to deal with reality. I decided that my best move was to try to stay ahead of the crashing media industry wave.

After I put out some feelers in the spring of 2013, a recruiter from the company that publishes *Vogue* called me. *Vogue* is best known as the world's leading fashion magazine, but it has also published some of the world's most celebrated writers, from Gloria Steinem to Ernest Hemingway. Because it was one of the few publications that could still attract significant ad revenue, it was also one of the world's most financially stable magazines. The staff is divided into two teams: the editors who work on the fashion stories and those who work on the feature stories. The job the recruiter was calling about involved working primarily with the latter team. During one of the several chats we had, the recruiter told me that she had read an essay I had published in *New York* several years earlier about my illness and said she admired it.

I believed her comment was sincere, but at the same time, I wondered if she might be fishing for information about my health status. It's not uncommon for people living with long-term illnesses to experience workplace discrimination. Disability claims are among the most reported types of complaints filed with the Equal Employment Opportunity Commission.

I told the recruiter that I appreciated the compliment and left it at that. The truth is, I did appreciate what she said, and if she had been looking for clues about my health, I wouldn't blame her. I might have done the same thing myself. In fact, I had been asking myself related ethical questions: Is it fair to take a new job without disclosing that I have a chronic illness? What if I get sick again and can't perform my duties? I decided that because I was in remission and didn't require any special accommodations, I had no obligation to talk about my health.

I also chose not to address my condition for another reason: Because I had been working at *New York* when I was diagnosed, just about all of my coworkers knew about my illness. In some ways, that was a burden. As much as I appreciated their questions about how I was doing and their sympathetic looks, those gestures could make me feel scrutinized. I didn't want to be the colleague with cancer; I just wanted to be a colleague.

Once you tell people you have cancer, you can't untell them. At a new job with new coworkers, I could have a fresh start.

13.

AFTER A FIRST-ROUND interview with a senior editor at *Vogue,* I was set to interview with Anna Wintour. Anna is rightly celebrated as the greatest editor in *Vogue*'s history and one of the greatest magazine editors, period. She is also known for being intimidating.

The obvious first question was what I should wear. Several days before my meeting, Didi and I discussed the matter. I said I was going to be a "words guy, not a fashion guy," and therefore could wear whatever I liked. The faded jeans and ratty T-shirts I wore at *New York* were obviously not in order, but a basic suit would be fine. Besides, why would I spend the money on a new suit when this was just an interview?

Didi, who had worked at a women's fashion magazine, told me as politely as she could that I was insane. My suits were boxy, baggy, and dated, she said. They made me look like David Byrne in *Stop Making Sense,* only three decades too late. It was true that I was going to be a "words" person, but it was going to be at a fashion magazine. I would be a fool not to dress appropriately for the interview. To put it in terms I could understand, she said that wearing one of my old suits would be like going to a Yankees tryout in a Red Sox uniform. That clicked. We made an emergency trip to Barneys and bought me a new suit, shirt, tie, and shoes. The bill came to more than half of our monthly mortgage payment.

The interview with Anna went well. She was warm and easygoing. It was actually more of a chat than an interview. I think she trusted at that point that I was capable of doing the job; this was mainly a chance to see if she and I would get along. Remarkably, I passed the test and was offered the position. Did she glance at my suit and shoes and seem to approve, or was that my imagination? I'll never know.

14.

AT MY *NEW YORK* magazine going-away party, Adam and some of my other colleagues said the sorts of lovely things people say on such occasions, and I did the same in return.

Honestly, I felt I should have thanked them more than they thanked me. Never mind how accepting and supportive everyone had been about my illness; it was the best, most rewarding job I'd had.

As a parting gesture, my colleagues gave me a present. The section of the magazine I had overseen was called "The Strategist," and the people who worked on it with me used to tease me for having a fatherly vibe. The gift was a fly-fishing rod. It was engraved with the words STRAT DAD.

15.

IT TOOK ME a while to fit in at *Vogue*. In one of my first meetings with Anna, she asked me to check on "the Horst story." She was referring to a piece about the legendary fashion photographer Horst P. Horst, only I hadn't heard of him and thought she said "horse." Naturally, I nodded, as if I knew what she was talking about, and figured it out later. During my first year at the magazine, when the invitation list for the famed Met Gala was being compiled, I asked one of the women in charge if editors like me were invited. She laughed.

Eventually, though, I found my groove. My colleagues and I published first-rate fashion spreads, feature stories, profiles, and essays and helped transition the publication from a print-only product to a multiplatform enterprise with a large web, social media, and video presence. Despite not being invited to the Met Gala, I did meet movie stars, politicians, rock stars, and athletes.

Because *Vogue*'s parent company, Condé Nast, was slow to recognize the importance of the internet, there was a lot of catching up to do to help bring the magazine into the digital era. That work was some of the most interesting I did at the magazine. We were helping to usher an iconic brand into the future, and from a careerist point of view, it helped me gain at least some experience in digital media. In my first year there, *Vogue* won the National Magazine Award for General Excellence, and two years later, it took home an even bigger prize, Magazine of the Year, which is given for a publication's print and nonprint work. I was proud to be part of that effort.

Because I remained in remission the entire time I was at *Vogue,* the issue of my illness never came up. Still, it could be uncomfortable to work there with a quasi-secret disease. Not that I feared anyone finding out (I'm sure they would have been lovely about it) or that I wanted anyone to know (the anonymity, as I noted, was a relief). But I felt as though I was hiding something. When you have a serious illness, you're damned if you tell people and damned if you don't.

Whenever people hear that I worked at *Vogue,* they ask me what I think of Anna. The answer is: I like her very much. She is a once-in-a-generation fashion visionary and whip smart. She has helped raise hundreds of millions of dollars for the Metropolitan Museum of Art, AIDS charities, and other causes. I also liked her direct, no-nonsense management style. She has a clear vision of what she wants and tells you exactly what that is. To me, that's fair. On occasion, I did see her speak to someone in a way you could describe as tough. But I've worked for any number of men who did the same or worse, and no one called them out on it.

Anna is also funnier than people know. One day on my way back to the *Vogue* offices from lunch, I was walking down the street in the expensive suit I had worn to my interview, licking an enormous Mister Softee chocolate-vanilla-swirl ice cream cone, when I ran into Anna walking with Amal Clooney. I thought that Anna would be horrified. Instead, she just smiled in a way that seemed to say, "Oh, Jon," as though I were a misbehaving puppy too hopeless to be embarrassed by.

16.

DIDI AND I, meanwhile, were at war. The good feelings we had managed to establish for a time had drained away, not because of any one issue or incident but because of the steady grinding together of misaligned marital tectonic plates. Our three main modes of communication were not speaking, bickering, and screaming at each other. We fought at home, we fought on the street, we fought at other people's dinner parties. The tension between us was so apparent at a friend's one night that he asked me, sympathetically, if we'd rather just leave. We barely hugged or held hands. Date nights didn't help, nor did any other purported self-help fixes.

We became the worst versions of ourselves. If Didi had been cold and distant before, now she was subarctic. If I had been condescending and controlling, I was now a flat-out asshole. About the best thing you could say for us is that we didn't fight in front of A.J. and Oscar. When they were present, we did our best to get along.

The Hollywood version of a couple going through cancer treatment together is all about unwavering devotion and appreciation. Our story wasn't like that.

Didi and I are hardly the only couple to experience problems brought on by a serious medical issue. Research on the subject shows that people who receive a cancer diagnosis are disproportionately depressed, anxious, angry, and irritable. They may feel physically unwell or experience issues regarding their life's purpose or their identity, all of which can create emotional distance between them and their spouse or partner and interfere with intimacy.

I checked most, if not all, of those boxes. And in addition to the caregiver burden effects Didi was experiencing, my illness had awakened one of her darkest fears, the fear of losing someone close to her. It was like touching the third rail of her psyche.

When you take your wedding vows, you agree to support each other in sickness and in health. But most of us are young and naive when we make that promise, and in any case, it's an abstraction. The boxer Mike Tyson famously said, "Everyone has a plan until they get punched in the mouth." In our marriage, cancer was the punch, and after ten years of living with it, we were stumbling around the ring.

In September 2013, Didi and I were running errands and the kids were home with a babysitter. Neither of us remembers what started it (the first law of marital thermodynamics states that the biggest fights often begin over the most trivial things), but before we knew it, we were sparring, then exchanging jabs, then throwing verbal haymakers on the corner of Astor Place and Lafayette Street. We were the couple other people tried not to stare at.

Soon, we were having the same fight we had had a thousand times before, the conflict I had come to think of as our Forever Fight: Didi didn't care that I was sick versus I expected too much from her. Only this time, we took things to a deeper, darker level. The fact that I didn't feel that Didi was sufficiently upset about my diagnosis led me to accuse her of not caring about me at all, ever. The fact that I felt that way, despite all she had been doing to keep me, herself, and the kids happy, led her to counterpunch with the idea that I was impossible to please. Seemingly, every issue we've ever had with each other, large and small, resurfaced. She was heartless, I was needy. I interrupted too much, she was constantly late. I mansplained, she didn't listen. We fought about how we fought: I was lawyerly, she was mean.

We traded blow after blow, each of us trying to gain the advantage, neither of us succeeding. Finally, after more than an hour, we stopped. We didn't resolve the fight so much as run out of gas. The bout ended in an ugly, unsatisfying draw.

The next morning, exhausted and punch drunk, we decided to see a couples counselor. Try as we might to work out our problems on our own, it was obvious that we were in over our heads. As individuals, we had managed to keep ourselves afloat reasonably well since my diagnosis, but as a couple, we were drowning.

17.

WE WERE LUCKY enough to work with a therapist, Dr. Hilary Weinger, whom we both liked and respected. Didi found Hilary, as she preferred we call her, through a friend. That woman and her husband had worked with Hilary after he had been diagnosed with cancer.

With curly black hair and an easy smile, Hilary is equal parts steel-trap smart, cheerful, and caring. She is roughly the same age as we are and has children about the same ages as A.J. and Oscar. Like Didi and me, she lives in Manhattan and raised her kids here. It turned out that we have other mutual friends.

At first, Didi and I treated therapy like a courtroom, each of us seeking to make the case to Hilary that he or she was right and the other person was wrong. We initially applied that approach to just about everything we discussed, but Hilary steered us toward a different dynamic, one in which she encouraged us to do our best to work together to resolve our differences. She encouraged us to listen, truly listen, to the other person's point of view and consider it honestly before reflexively opposing it. Once we agreed to do that, or at least to try, we began to make progress.

In our early sessions, we mainly talked about the Forever Fight. When I told Hilary I was angry at Didi for not being more outwardly upset by my illness and withdrawing from me emotionally, Hilary suggested that her behavior might be related to losing her father and her fear of having to go through that kind of pain again. It wasn't an idea Didi and I hadn't thought of, but hearing Hilary say it validated it. It made me feel less angry toward Didi, and it made Didi feel less guilty about not being more visibly upset.

When we talked about my expecting too much from Didi, Hilary helped us see how that desire traced back to cancer. When life deals you a nasty hand, it's hard not to feel that you deserve special treatment. Because Didi was the person closest to me, I wanted her to provide that. That was reasonable up to a point, Hilary pointed out, but expecting too much from her was making her feel suffocated. Instead, she suggested that I trust in the ideas that (a) I was lovable and (b) Didi loved me. Those thoughts helped me reset my expectations to a more realistic level, which then helped Didi feel less pressured.

Eventually, Didi and I came to see that while cancer had caused its own set of difficulties, it had also shone a light on preexisting issues we'd been pretending weren't there. Cancer hadn't created our problems so much as exposed them.

Hilary also helped Didi and me confront some of our deepest fears about our relationship, fears that were contributing to the distance between us. She helped me see that I was afraid of Didi's leaving me, to then have to face cancer, and die, alone. She helped me see that I was afraid that no one else would ever want to be with me if Didi and I split up, because who would want to date someone with an incurable disease? She helped Didi see that she felt trapped by the idea that she couldn't leave me even if she wanted to because she was afraid she would feel like a monster for abandoning a sick spouse. Her bringing those fears into the open helped quiet them.

On the whole, couples therapy was a grueling and humbling process. It's not easy to admit your darkest fears or cop to bad habits you've had for decades. But in fits and starts, Didi and I began to do that, to see ourselves and each other in turn.

Gradually, the ice storm we'd been experiencing on and off for years began to pass. The peaks of our relationship became a little higher, and the valleys became a little less low. That fresh glimmer of hope sparked a spirit of optimism about our relationship that encouraged us to keep working on it. We had a long way to go, but at least we could see a path forward. Cancer had nearly torn apart our marriage, but by pushing us to the brink, it had also brought us to a place where we might be able to mend it.

After a little more than a year of weekly fifty-minute sessions, Hilary encouraged us to stop our therapy and try to work things out on our own, using what we'd learned from working with her. To be honest, Didi and I were afraid to leave. If nothing else, Hilary had helped keep the peace between us, and neither of us wanted to go back to combat. But Hilary assured us that we were moving in the right direction and could manage our relationship ourselves. If we had trouble, we could always come back, she said. Cautiously, we agreed.

18.

A.J. AND OSCAR were eleven and six. After passing through a princess phase and a horse phase, A.J. had developed an interest in singing and acting, joining her grade school choral group, the Songbirds, and performing as Liesl in *The Sound of Music* at a neighborhood children's theater. Lots of parents get emotional when they see their kids perform, but I was wrecked. I don't know what the exact circuitry involved entailed, but A.J.'s performances seemed to trigger my fear of dying. It's as if my limbic system were saying, *This is making me happy. I do not want it to end.*

On Saturday mornings, Oscar and I would go to our local YMCA, something A.J. and I had also done when she was younger. I've always loved to swim, and I enjoyed passing along that tradition. Swimming together, particularly when the kids were little and dependent on me for their survival, is also a powerful bonding experience. Some of my happiest times with my kids were spent in that pool.

Remember the concerns I'd had about A.J.'s health? Those worries extended to her emotional well-being, and to Oscar's. If either of them seemed sad, scared, or anxious for no apparent reason, Didi and I would wonder: Do they somehow know I'm sick? Is it making them upset? Could they sense our marital problems? Whenever either child was struggling emotionally, we felt doubly bad. We felt for them, and we worried that we might be at least partly responsible.

As much as I worried about anything, I worried about leaving A.J. and Oscar fatherless. If there is anything hardwired into parents of the human species, it is to protect and provide for their offspring. To be unable to do so would feel like an unforgivable failure.

My fears weren't unwarranted. Research shows that children who lose a parent frequently experience anxiety and depression. They may withdraw from friends and struggle in school.

Just as I worried about leaving my kids without a father, I worried about leaving Didi without a husband. The so-called widowhood effect, when one spouse dies shortly after his or her partner does, is commonly thought to apply mainly to older couples. But a study published in 2023 in the science and medical journal *PLOS ONE* found that younger people are even more at risk. The researchers hypothesized that the loss of a spouse may be more traumatic for a younger person because it's less expected. In addition to experiencing higher rates of premature death, spouses who lose a partner are disproportionately prone to anxiety, depression, post-traumatic stress disorder, and loneliness, itself a risk factor for other illnesses.

Among its other charms, cancer is a sea of worries. When you're not worried about yourself, you're worried that you're hurting someone else.

19.

OVER THE YEARS, my parents, my sisters and brother, their spouses, and my nephews and nieces have all done events to raise money for multiple myeloma research. In that way and others too numerous to count, they have been an unflagging source of support.

My brother is a runner, but until the spring of 2014, he had never run a marathon. That April, at age fifty-one, Andy ran the Boston Marathon to raise awareness and money for the Multiple Myeloma Research Foundation.

On the day of the event, a group of our family and friends met at Andy's house in Newton, Massachusetts, and walked to a nearby viewing point between miles twenty and twenty-one on the infamous Heartbreak Hill. By the time Andy reached that spot, he indeed looked broken. To help spur him on, we gave him some orange wedges, and he and I exchanged a hug. He finished the race in 5:08:04. (The winner that year was the legendary Eritrean-born American runner Meb Keflezighi, who posted a time of 2:08:37.) Andy was so sore the next day that he had to shimmy down the stairs on his ass. For two days after that, he could descend only backward. All told, he raised $45,000, primarily through Facebook and from family members, coworkers, friends, and friends of friends.

A few days after the race, I sent an email to Jen, Tina, and Andy and copied Didi: "They say all a person really wants in life is to know he's loved, especially by his family. Mission accomplished, people! Thank you for a day I will obviously never forget. Extra thanks, of course, to the guy who did the jogging."

Andy wrote back, "I am basking in the glow of one of the best days of my life. The emotion and joy were worth every step."

Then Didi weighed in: "Andy, everything you've done has moved us so much. And someday (soon), the kiddies will also know the full scope of your deed. And—as if it were possible—they'll love you even more."

20.

IN MAY 2014, I had a routine checkup in Boston with Dr. Richardson. In his ongoing effort to help me stay ahead of my illness, he raised the subject of my frozen stem cells. The fact that I had survived myeloma for more than ten years without having a stem cell transplant was terrific, he said. Nevertheless, I might still need a transplant someday, and he was concerned about the viability of my frozen cells after so many years. It was a good problem to have, but it was still a problem. He suggested that I speak to my doctors at Mount Sinai, where my stem cells were being stored, to get their opinion.

If my cells were no longer usable, Dr. Richardson said, he could "recollect" me—that is, do another stem cell harvest. But that procedure would be more involved than it was the first time. Because my disease was more advanced, I would have to have a round of chemotherapy first, to be certain there was either no disease in my cells or as little as possible. Dr. Richardson referred to the chemotherapy as "real chemotherapy," by which he meant treatment more difficult and debilitating than any of the treatments I'd had to date. Even after the chemotherapy, my stem cells, having been subjected to ten-plus years of my disease plus three rounds of radiation and RVD, would likely be less efficacious than my original stem cells would be, assuming that they were still viable.

If my original stem cells were, in fact, no longer viable, the other alternative, Dr. Richardson said, was what's called an allogeneic, as opposed to autologous, stem cell transplant. In an allogeneic transplant, the stem cells that are used are not yours but those of a donor. No matter how close a match the donor is, Dr. Richardson explained, an allogeneic transplant can be more effective than an autologous transplant but typically has more debilitating side effects. That said, the closer the match, the better, and the closest matches are generally one's siblings. If my sisters and brother were a match, that would make recollecting me less urgent. He recommended that I ask them to be tested.

Despite the fact that a standard blood draw is all that's required to determine if someone is a match, I hated to ask Jen, Tina, and Andy to do it. I was reluctant to put anyone out for anything having to do with my illness, and I definitely didn't want to force one of my sisters or my brother to potentially undergo a stem cell harvest. But because I had no choice, I sent them an email one afternoon explaining what was going on and asking them if they would be willing to be tested. Within an hour, they all replied that they'd be happy to help.

That turned out to be the easy part. Although the blood draws themselves were simple enough, none of my siblings' doctors was familiar with the precise test they needed to order, and a Keystone Cops routine ensued. Despite the fact that I had gotten the necessary information from Dr. Richardson's office and passed it along to Jen, Tina, and Andy, who in turn had forwarded it to their doctors, the correct tests still weren't ordered in every case and in some instances had to be redone. Even when the proper results were obtained, they sometimes weren't sent to Dr. Richardson's office or got lost on his end. Over the course of several months, dozens of emails, phone calls, and faxes were exchanged.

While that bureaucratic dance played out, I made an appointment with Dr. Jagannath. Since I had last seen him, Dr. Jagannath had left St. Vincent's and was now the director of the Center of Excellence for Multiple Myeloma at Mount Sinai. I had barely finished explaining why I had come to see him when he told me that he wasn't concerned about my stem cells. He had recently transplanted a patient of his using cells almost twice as old as mine, and the procedure had been a success, he said. There was no need to recollect me.

I was tremendously relieved. The phrase "real chemotherapy" had left an impression on me. Also, Jen, Tina, and Andy wouldn't have to donate their stem cells. We never did find out who was and wasn't a match; once I learned my own stem cells were still viable, we dropped the matter. That was just as well as far as I was concerned. The bureaucratic bungling turned out to be a blessing. No one would have to worry about donating someday.

21.

IN JUNE 2014, Didi and I decided to tell A.J. that I had cancer. She was eleven years old and about to graduate from elementary school. Something about that milestone seemed to prompt us. The best approach, we decided, was for me to find a moment when A.J. and I were alone and out of the house. We didn't want to create a dramatic "family meeting" moment or tell her in our apartment, where the memory of the conversation could linger. Because I was the directly affected party, it made sense for me to tell her. Dr. Gol had suggested that I keep my message short, then let A.J. ask any questions she might have; that way, she could take on as much or as little information as she was ready to.

And so on a Saturday afternoon, in a cab on our way to Bloomingdale's to buy A.J. her grade school graduation dress, I told her. What I said was "I have something to tell you. I have cancer. I've had it for a long time, since just after you were born. Right now, I'm totally healthy—you can see that with your own eyes—and my doctors expect to keep me that way for a long time. So now you know."

What A.J. said was "Well, that's a surprise." Then she asked why we hadn't told her sooner, and I explained that Didi and I had talked to a lot of people about it and decided it didn't make sense to tell a small child about something that wasn't an immediate problem and that she probably couldn't understand. She asked what kind of cancer I had.

She asked how I had found out I had it. She asked if I was really okay, and I assured her I was. Then I told her that I would always be happy to answer any questions she had or listen to any worries or fears. I reassured her again that I really was okay and promised that I would tell her the truth about my illness from that point on.

There was a little more back-and-forth over those same questions, and she asked, sweetly, if it was okay for her to tell her friends. But for the time being, that was it. As painful as the conversation was, it was also a relief. Secrets, even well-intentioned ones, can be heavy. Keeping my illness from A.J. and Oscar had been weighing on me and Didi for years. That burden, at least, had been lifted.

A short time later, I told Oscar. It came up, as it happened, the way I had thought it might have with A.J. When Oscar told me one day that he wanted to learn how to ski, I said that sounded great but I couldn't teach him myself. Then I told him why and repeated more or less the same speech I had given A.J. He asked some of the same questions A.J. had asked, and he seemed fairly unbothered.

Years later, when she was in her twenties, A.J. told me that she appreciated that we hadn't told her until we did. She said she wouldn't have gotten it when she was younger anyway, and it had kept her from having to worry. Oscar said he felt the same way.

A.J.'s graduation dress, by the way, was a midlength white cotton sundress with lace trim. She looked beautiful.

22.

IT'S UNCLEAR WHY, but later that summer, the drug I was on to control the diarrhea triggered by the Revlimid stopped working. I frequently had to rush to the bathroom again. I prayed that the subway wouldn't stop between stations for any length of time. I chose aisle seats for flights and movies so I could get up quickly if I needed to. I occasionally had to make excuses to leave meetings at *Vogue*, of all places, to race to the restroom.

I lived that way for the better part of a year. I lost twenty-five pounds. I was afraid that if I raised the issue with my doctors, I'd have to go off Revlimid. If living this way was the cost of realizing Revlimid's potentially life-extending benefits, I was willing to pay.

Then one day on my way to dinner with a friend, I found myself desperately needing to use the bathroom and almost had another accident. It was a wake-up call. The next day, I made an appointment to see my gastroenterologist. He suggested that I try a powdered form of cholestyramine that some of his patients had had success with. Mercifully, it worked. You dissolve a tablespoon of the powder into a glass of water first thing in the morning, drink it, then wait at least half an hour before you eat or drink anything else. From that point on, that's how I've started my day. Some people have coffee; I have cholestyramine.

23.

MY FRIENDS RANDY, Jeff, Eric, and I—the postcollegiate buddy-trip crew—along with our friend Ted, traveled to New Orleans that fall. Once again, we had a wonderful time—chargrilled oysters at the Acme Oyster House, a New Orleans Saints football game, and a live outdoor performance by a local Dixieland band were highlights—but on that trip, there was no escaping cancer.

On the night we arrived, I decided to take another chance on drinking and almost passed out from dehydration again, this time in a bar. Randy, Jeff, Eric, and Ted had to get me into a cab and take me back to our hotel, where I drank bottle after bottle of water and went to sleep. It was the first time my friends had seen a visible manifestation of my illness. I think it may have shaken them. I know it shook me. This time, there was no pretending that we were still in college or I didn't have cancer. There was no imagining that we were living in the past. There was just the too real present.

24.

FLY-FISHING IS EXPENSIVE, even more so if you like to travel to do it. To offset the cost of my angling adventures, I decided to try to write newspaper and magazine stories about them. I pitched an idea about bonefishing, a sport within the sport I hadn't yet tried, to an editor I knew and landed an assignment. I asked my friend and fishing buddy Tim if he'd like to come along, and we were off on a three-day excursion to South Andros Island in the Bahamas.

Bonefish are a thrill to catch. More like hunting than conventional angling, bonefishing isn't a chuck-your-line-in-the-water-and-pray type of deal. A guide leads you to a promising flat, where you stand on the casting deck of a small shallow-water skiff as he poles you, gondola style. (You might also wade into the water on foot.) Because bones' mirrored backs make them wickedly difficult to spot against the bottom of the sandy flats, it can take hours to locate one, and your guide will likely spot it before you do. With sharks and barracuda as their predators, bones spook at the first sign of a threat. Get too close or drop the cooler lid too loudly, and they're gone. It's no wonder that the species is known as the gray ghost.

When your guide finds a fish, he'll call out its position:

"Bonefish. Two o'clock. Twenty feet." You cast your fly just ahead of your target, ideally within a foot or two of its nose. With luck, your quarry sees it, gulps it down, and takes off. Before you can say "Fish on," your line is taut, your reel is whizzing, and your rod is bent in half.

Located about 150 miles southeast of Miami, South Andros is often referred to as the bonefishing capital of the world. Populated by just a few thousand laid-back folks and unmarred by large-scale resorts or casinos, the island is a *Gilligan*-esque haven of tiny airstrips, sleepy towns, and deserted beaches. Bonefish sometimes gather in such large numbers here that when they eat the shrimp and small crabs that are their primary diet, they can kick up so much sand that their "mudding" can be seen from a plane above. Three- to five-pound specimens are the most common, but ten- to fifteen-pound monsters are not unheard of.

On our first day of fishing, less than an hour after we'd shoved off into the clear turquoise waters of South Andros for the first time, our guide, Harlan "Harley" Sands, a hard-living, fun-loving fiftysomething Bahamian with a cache of stories about growing up on the mean streets of Nassau, zeroed in on a target.

"Bones coming at twelve o'clock," he said. "Get ready."

Tim, who was fishing first, pointed his rod toward that spot on the clock.

"A little to the right," Harlan said. "Forty feet and coming straight at us."

Tim spotted the fish Harlan pointed to, drew a bead on it, and made a cast.

"Short, man. Go again!"

Tim's next cast was on the money; the fish saw it and chased his fly.

"Set!" Harlan said.

The fish was hooked and took off across the flat, leaving a rooster tail of saltwater spray behind it. After the fish made two quick runs, Tim reeled it in, removed the hook from its lip, and released it. It was a good-size bone, not the biggest the world has seen but not the smallest, either.

But the speed! "Bahamian missile," Harlan said.

We were officially on the scoreboard.

As the morning wore on, Harlan would find a bone, Tim would catch it. Harlan would find a bone, Tim would catch it. Before long, Tim was spotting his own fish and bringing them to the boat.

After a period of flailing, I managed to put my fly in front of a fish, watched as he started to chase it, set the hook the moment he sucked it down, and reeled him in. He was a solid five-pounder, the biggest fish we'd caught so far. I felt a mix of shock and euphoria. Harlan recognized the condition instantly.

"That's right," he said. "You got the jones for the bones."

About our second day, the less said the better, and our third day began with a dry spell as well. At one point, Tim stepped down from the casting deck a bit before his allotted time was up. "All you, buddy," he said to me.

His thoughtfulness cost him. Within moments of my stepping up, our guide called out a fish. I made a cast and hooked up. While a few of the bones we'd caught had made decent runs, none had lived up to the species' hell-bent-for-leather reputation.

This one did. In what seemed like a second, he was fifty yards away . . . seventy-five . . . a hundred . . . he took me deep into the backing of my line, and right when I was beginning to fear he'd snap it and light out for Bora Bora, he eased up. I reeled like mad, trying to recover line while I had the chance.

When I had my quarry within a few feet of the boat, I could see he was a healthy four-pounder with a pretty turquoise back and cobalt tail. Then he took off and did it all over again.

On that final run, when he appeared as just a tiny swoosh of spray on the horizon, when the sun sparkled off that immaculate white sand flat, when my reel was screaming and my heart rate redlining—well, that's bonefishing. Eventually, I landed him. That night, I had a dream about catching that fish. I've had the same dream dozens of times since.

The views on the flight home were some of the prettiest I've seen. The ocean was a giant pane of aquamarine glass, and the late-afternoon sun turned a skyful of cumulus clouds a shade of coral worthy of Monet. It occurred to me: Would I have done this trip if I had never gotten sick? Would I have had the same appetite for new experiences? The same sense of urgency? Although it pains me to grant cancer credit for anything good, I knew the answer. Being sick has motivated me to try new things.

The following week, I celebrated my fiftieth birthday. Didi threw a party for me at a faux speakeasy on Manhattan's Lower East Side. Many of my friends and family members were there, and we ate, drank, and danced until well after midnight. I am aware that many people dread that midlife milestone, but I was thrilled by it. I was alive. I was relatively well. I was seeing my kids grow up. Fifty wasn't a burden; it was a gift.

25.

FOR A TIME after we had stopped seeing Hilary, Didi and I had maintained the momentum we had built while working with her. But after a year and a half or so, we had begun to backslide. Instead of patiently trying to understand where the other person was coming from and why, we reverted to our reactionary annoyance when the other person did anything we didn't like. Instead of doing our best to avoid doing the things that drove the other person crazy, we went back to our old stubborn, defensive habits. As our empathy ebbed, the ice storm roared back in. In April 2016, we returned to therapy.

For the first six months of our second stint, Didi and I slogged along, taking one step forward, then two steps back. If we weren't getting any worse, we weren't getting any better, either.

Then, on October 25, 2016, Didi and I went out to dinner to celebrate our nineteenth wedding anniversary. At the restaurant, a new place in the West Village we had been wanting to try, we picked at our food, didn't talk much, and avoided eye contact. We each tried to generate some warmth, but to no avail. As soon as we were done with dessert and coffee, we asked the server for the check. Our anniversary only made the grim state of our relationship more plain to see.

After Didi and I put A.J. and Oscar to bed, we got into another brutal, all-hours row. This time, we were truly on the brink. We were tired of fighting and tired of being miserable. The status quo was no longer an option. We both felt we either needed to fix things once and for all or split up.

At our next session with Hilary, when we told her about the fight, she said we basically had three choices: We could end the marriage, change the terms of it, or try to save it. Whatever we chose to do, she said, she could help us, but deciding that would help her figure out how to best proceed. It made for the kind of dramatic therapist's office moment scene you see in the movies but rarely in real life.

When Didi and I both said we wanted to save our marriage, the weather in the room shifted. Something about that decision was transformative. As awful a place as we were in—and it was indeed awful—that decision was a pivotal first step in getting us back into the spirit of working together to resolve our differences. The process was still going to be long and difficult, and it wasn't at all clear if it would work. But as Didi pointed out after that session, we at least had a clear common purpose. Just hearing each other say we wanted to try was helpful. It was a mutual expression, however complicated and fragile, of commitment, possibly even love.

Slowly, Didi and I started to move forward again. The progress was far from smooth. Issues came to light that were extremely painful, issues neither of us were proud of. Each of us left more than one session feeling wounded and angry and wondering if our marriage could, in fact, be saved. But the more we chipped away at the roots of our difficulties—the same fundamental problems we had discussed when we had seen Hilary the first time—the better we began to get along. Our relationship, while far from perfect, was improving again.

The following spring, Hilary suggested that we were ready to move on. As before, we were hesitant. As before, she assured us that we would be okay.

26.

IN SEPTEMBER 2016, I had lunch with my friend Mark. Mark and I had worked together at *Men's Journal* magazine and had remained close friends. For a number of years, we had played together in a poker game he regularly hosted at the apartment he shared with his wife and two young children, but that game had eventually disbanded when Mark, the other players, and I had disappeared into the black hole of parenthood and careerdom.

Recently, however, Mark and his wife had separated, and he had moved into his own apartment. I, meanwhile, had been looking for another diversion from illness and the uncertainty it brings—something other than fishing, basically, that could distract me. It had occurred to me that a non-physical activity could be useful. If somewhere down the line I wound up physically disabled, I wanted to have a hobby of the mind, not the body.

The first edition of our reborn poker game was held at Mark's bachelor apartment in Harlem that November. Mark and I reenlisted several players from the original group and recruited a number of new participants, mostly present and former colleagues from the media business and their friends and acquaintances.

We don't play for high stakes. It's more like a book club than a casino; we get together to hang out and talk as much as we do to win or lose money. Everyone brings a six-pack, we order some pizzas, and we talk about everything from politics to sports, books, and movies (unless you have a *lot* of time, do not ask my friend Scott about *The Beatles: Get Back*) to our spouses, girlfriends and boyfriends, and children. More than thirty people are included on the email invitation that goes out. We play on Monday nights, and on any given week, six to twelve of us show up. We mostly play no-limit Texas Hold 'Em and Pot-Limit Omaha, and we split into two tables if necessary.

Fairly early on, we started a tradition of giving one another unapologetically dumb nicknames. Because he runs the game, Mark is "El Jefe." Owing to my habit of whining when I lose or even just don't win enough, I have been dubbed "J Miz." For the obvious reasons, our friend John Campbell is "Soup." Certain bets have nicknames, too, although it's probably best I don't explain the etymology of the Duck Dick. Because we initially played on Mark's kitchen table, which was made of mango tree wood, we call the game "The Mango."

As I write this, we have been playing every week for more than eight years, or more than four hundred weeks, almost without exception (when the pandemic hit, we switched to playing virtually, using an app called PokerBros to facilitate the game and Zooming to socialize). Some of our kids sometimes play with us. Several players have had kids since the game started. My devotion to the game is such that I have been known to spend the day in Boston receiving cancer treatment, then fly home and go straight to the poker table from the airport.

At one point after the pandemic began, Mark wrote a story for *Esquire* magazine about the Mango. In it, he said, "I keep a scrupulous running tally of weekly wins and losses (I'm up overall, thank you very much), but of course it isn't the money that matters. This game, for me—for us—is a lifeline, an anchor in tough and turbulent times, a reliable weekly six-hour moment to let it all go and just be."

That's exactly right.

27.

ONE EVENING AROUND that time, I was riding the subway home from work when I found myself involuntarily shaking my head. The same thing has happened to me a number of times since. Every now and then, usually when I'm doing something mindless, like watching TV or chopping vegetables for dinner, it suddenly occurs to me, for no apparent reason, that I have cancer, and I shake my head as if to say, *I can't believe it*. *I still* can't believe it. It's like the way I shook my head when Oscar was born, only a bad shake, not a good one.

Sometimes our lives, even though they're ours, still aren't believable. They're somehow both real and uncanny.

28.

THAT WINTER, I passed the five-year mark of my Revlimid-induced remission. I was aware of the milestone but chose not to celebrate it.

While I maintain that I'm not religious in the going-to-temple sense of the word, I was starting to wonder if maybe superstition is actually my faith. Maybe kissing the back of my knuckles is my Hail Mary. Maybe the stuffed tiger I keep by my bedside is my rosary beads. Not that my feelings on the matter are at all consistent. Sometimes kissing my hands or keeping a stuffed animal next to my bed feels like the most sensible and important thing I could possibly do to stay well, and other times, it feels as though I'm insane. In any case, I chose to pretend that nothing meaningful was happening when I crossed the five-year remission threshold. My "logic" was, don't poke the bear.

I noticed something else at around that time: When you've been living with a medical condition for years, especially if you don't have any outward signs of your illness, friends and family can sometimes treat you as though you're not really sick or you've been cured. Eventually, some people stop asking how you are, and others disappear from your life altogether. There's even a term for it: "cancer ghosting."

That's all understandable. Being around someone who's sick can be anxiety inducing and depressing; a kind of caring fatigue can set in. With enough time, even cancer can become wallpaper. At the same time, those of us living with long-term illnesses can't walk away from our conditions. We can't ghost ourselves.

29.

I MENTIONED THAT Didi and I had taken out life insurance policies shortly before A.J. was born and nine months before I was diagnosed with cancer. That was the fortunate part of our life insurance story.

The unfortunate part came in January 2017 when I received a letter from MetLife, our policy carrier, indicating that it was getting out of certain aspects of the life insurance business, including the one involving our coverage.

For the previous fourteen years, Didi and I had had so-called term life policies—each with a twenty-year term, each worth $1 million should we die. The premiums were $790 per year for me and $640 for Didi. (Because men, on average, die earlier than women, life insurance is generally more expensive for them.)

Now we were being told that we had a choice: Keep the policies until their terms ended, six years hence, or convert them to so-called whole life policies now. If we converted the policies now, we would not have to undergo medical tests to qualify for the new type of coverage. If we didn't convert now, we would essentially be starting from scratch in 2023, and at that point, we would have to undergo medical tests to get a new policy. Given my health status, it was unclear if I would be able to get a new policy at all, and if I was able to get one, it was sure to be tremendously expensive. What Didi and I decided to do was keep her term policy (because she was healthy, she could likely get a new policy at a reasonable cost when it expired) but convert mine to whole life.

A $1 million whole life policy would have cost me $11,516 annually, almost fifteen times the cost of my previous coverage. Because that was out of the question, we decided to reduce my coverage to $250,000. Even so, my new whole life policy costs $2,879, almost four times the price of my previous policy, for one-fourth of the coverage. To offset the extra expense, we reduced Didi's term coverage from $1 million to $500,000, reducing the cost of her coverage to $370 per year.

Because of the not insignificant chance that I would die prematurely, I also elected to buy additional life insurance through *Vogue*'s parent company during its open enrollment period that year. That policy, which covered three times my salary if I died, set me back another $3,000 per year. Didi and I automatically had a basic amount of life insurance through our employers, but we weren't comfortable with that level of coverage, given my circumstances.

Although I appreciated the fact that MetLife had offered us a chance to convert our term life policies without having to undergo a medical exam, it was essentially forcing us to pay a lot more money for a lot less coverage. The original letter the company sent announcing the change it was making began "Dear Valued Customer." I should have known at that moment I was in trouble.

When I had worked at *New York* magazine, the company had offered disability insurance as part of employees' basic benefits package. In 2011, the company that provided that coverage offered *New York* employees the opportunity to buy supplemental coverage for an additional fee, no questions asked. When I had asked a friend who was in finance if he thought I should take advantage of that offer, he had pointed out that if I were to become disabled, the financial impact could be catastrophic. If I died, I wouldn't be earning any money, but I wouldn't be incurring any expenses, either. If I were alive and so sick I couldn't work, on the other hand, I might have a double whammy of no income and exorbitant expenses. I bought the supplemental insurance. That coverage costs me another $1,303.93 per year.

I'm not crying poverty. I'm lucky to have the money I have and to be able to afford insurance. But any way you look at it, having cancer is expensive.

30.

AT *NEW YORK* magazine, one of my fellow editors was Joanna Coles. Joanna had gone on to become the chief content officer of Hearst Magazines, the publisher of *Esquire, Elle, Harper's Bazaar,* and other titles. When a position opened at Hearst in the summer of 2017, Joanna called to see if I was interested.

The opening in question was an executive-level job that involved recruiting high-level editorial talent and launching new magazines. It was a bigger opportunity than I'd had a shot at before, and hiring people and starting new publications were two of my favorite things to do. I was fifty-two years old. If everything went right, it could be my final job, a nice coda to my magazine career. The interview process went well, and by August, I was negotiating the details of an offer with David Carey, the president of Hearst Magazines.

At the time, Didi, A.J., Oscar, and I were on Fire Island, the summer vacation destination off Long Island. The night I finalized my deal with Carey, A.J. went out with friends.

Half an hour past her curfew, when she hadn't come home, I sent her a cheeky text: "Hey, GRLLL! 'Sup?" Only I didn't send it to her. I sent it to Carey.

I panicked. At best, he would see me as a bumbler; at worst, God knows what. But texting again to explain that the message had been meant for my fourteen-year-old daughter didn't seem like such a great idea, either. Rather than call further attention to my stupidity, I decided not to do anything. Sometimes, inaction is the best action.

David, bless him, never said a word.

On my last day at *Vogue*, my colleagues threw me a party with champagne and macarons and a mock issue of the magazine with me on the cover (a standard magazine trope). It was a lovely gesture, and I was sad to leave. At the same time, I was excited to start something new.

31.

IN MY FIRST year at Hearst, I helped hire new editors in chief and design directors for several of the company's magazines—*Men's Health, Women's Health, Cosmopolitan, Elle*—and began developing new publications. In the course of my recruiting work, I also spoke to scores of talented and experienced people, including a number of former colleagues, who were out of work and had been for prolonged periods of time. It was like having a grim front-row seat to the death of the magazine business. It also had an eerie feeling of foreshadowing.

The most promising of the new publications I was working on was a project involving Jimmy Buffett. As it happened, Joanna Coles knew Buffett's wife, and she helped us secure a meeting with him and the executive who ran his businesses.

Buffett and I immediately hit it off. He and one of my

former bosses were friends, and he was every bit as warm, openhearted, and friendly as his public image would have you believe. But that wasn't what fostered our connection; we bonded over fly-fishing.

Buffett's love of sitting on a beach sipping a certain frozen cocktail may be more widely known, but he was also a passionate angler. An experienced pilot, he'd had a Grumman HU-16 Albatross "flying boat" seaplane custom outfitted for the sport (rod rack, fly-tying bench, etc.) and made regular trips to the Caribbean and Central and South America to fish out of it. He would scout a promising ocean flat, one that had very likely never been fished by any human, land the Albatross, hop out, and have at it. I would say it was a fly-fisher's dream, but frankly, it was beyond anything any angler would have allowed themselves to imagine.

The first time we met, Buffett and I talked about that plane and his adventures on it for maybe twenty minutes until it became apparent that we were boring the rest of the folks in the meeting. He invited me to come along with him one day to fish from the Albatross.

With a number of others, I began to work on the Hearst collaboration. I also started dreaming of a trip on that plane.

32.

IN THE SPRING of 2018, I went to Dr. Gruenstein's office for my monthly infusion of Zometa, the bone-strengthening drug I had been taking for roughly ten years. But when I arrived, Dr. Gruenstein told me about a new drug called Xgeva (generic name denosumab). Xgeva served the same function as Zometa, he said, but it was given as an injection, not intravenously. Instead of taking an hour or more to work, it takes only minutes. That was its main advantage compared to Zometa. Its disadvantages were that it could cause a drop in vitamin D level (but I could take a simple over-the-counter supplement for that) and it carried a slightly higher risk of developing osteonecrosis of the jaw. Because I had been on Zometa for so long without experiencing ONJ, I decided to make the switch.

33.

LATER THAT SAME spring, after almost twenty years of working with her, I decided to end my therapy with Dr. Gol. That didn't mean I was by any means immune to being upset, angry, or sad; it just meant that I felt I could handle what life brought my way, good and bad, with a livable degree of equanimity. She had taught me the word *equanimity*.

On the previous occasions when I had talked about leaving therapy, Dr. Gol had suggested that I stay, that I still had work to do. But this time, she agreed that I was in a good place. She encouraged me to go through an ending phase of therapy in which accomplishments and unresolved issues are shared. Although that process is considered to be an important part of therapy, it takes time, and I felt impatient. Instead, we had a few wind-down sessions, then finished our work together.

At the end of our final session, when we said our goodbyes, I was emotional but not overly so. I teared up when we hugged, but what I felt more than anything was a deep sense of stability. Dr. Gol radiated that herself, on that day and always.

As I turned to leave, she said to me, "The door is always open."

When I had started seeing Dr. Gol, just about anything could bother me. When I left, I felt as though I could cope with cancer, work problems, marital troubles, issues with my kids, and more. I felt like a more resilient human being.

Unlike my medical doctors, Dr. Gol didn't save my life; she just made it infinitely better.

34.

I HAVE ALWAYS liked to travel. One of my fondest childhood memories is of a trip my family and I took to Disney World. I loved the Haunted Mansion and Splash Mountain, and my parents bought me a Goofy watch that blew my little eight-year-old mind (Goofy was my favorite character, not Mickey; make of that what you will). Then there was an epic two-week road trip from the Grand Canyon to Seattle (cut short in Portland due to unconscionably bad teenage behavior by myself and two of my siblings but still wonderful somehow, at least in my sepia-tinted memory) and a three-part pilgrimage to Gettysburg, Colonial Williamsburg, and Hershey, Pennsylvania.

As the child of a mother and father who were touring musicians born and raised abroad, Didi was virtually born with a passport in her hand. When she was four, her mother put her onto a plane from New York to Buenos Aires by herself to visit her grandmother.

As parents, Didi and I have tried to pass on our fondness for traveling to A.J. and Oscar, and in the summer of 2018, we took a family trip to Iceland.

The trip didn't get off to the best start. Flying, like exercise and drinking, can cause dehydration, all the more on long flights. On the way from New York to Reykjavík, I was sitting across the aisle from Didi and the kids when I suddenly felt woozy. When I came to, I was lying in the aisle with a doctor and flight attendant reviving me.

Anytime I feel as though I've upset or put out Didi or the kids because of my illness, I feel guilty, and in that case, I was worried that I had terrified them. At first, it seemed that my concern was unnecessary. Once it was clear that I was all right, they all laughed. Part of it was nervous laughter; by laughing, they were making the situation okay. Part of it was embarrassed laughter. What kid isn't mortified by their parents' public gaffes? And part of it was laughter laughter. On some level, seeing their husband and father tip over and conk out in the aisle of a plane played like physical comedy. But the truth is that the incident was scary and left us all a little uneasy. As a parent, you want to feel like a rock. Lying in the aisle of that plane, I felt I was starting to crack.

The rest of the trip, fortunately, was amazing. Over the course of our five-day stay, we swam in the Blue Lagoon and applied Instagram-friendly mud masks. We hiked on otherworldly black sand beaches and traversed centuries-old glaciers. We climbed behind enormous cascading waterfalls. We toured historic cathedrals. We ate locally baked bread and enjoyed homemade ice cream at a dairy farm. We went puffin watching, and in the souvenir shop afterward, Oscar got an adorable puffin hat.

Because I am both a cheapskate and a cancer patient who may or may not be obsessed with family togetherness, the four of us stayed in the same room, with the kids sleeping on cots. We ate breakfast in bed together and watched the World Cup on TV.

On the last day of our stay, Oscar and I hiked a steep trail that wound its way up the face of a mountain on the outskirts of Reykjavík. When we got as close to the summit as we could without needing rock-climbing gear, we stopped to catch our breath, take in the view, and pat ourselves on the

back. Oscar had undergone some preteen challenges the previous year and had just come through them before we had
left for the trip. I had overcome my own share of adversity. It
was not lost on me that he and I had just climbed a mountain
together.

Trips like that with my kids are fantastic, and I'm grateful
for all of them. But since I got sick, I've found that just playing Uno, watching *Family Guy*, making waffles, doing crossword puzzles, going grocery shopping, or taking a walk with
Didi, A.J., and Oscar are every bit as enjoyable. If anything,
I'm at my most content doing nothing at all with them.

Illness simplifies your needs. It purifies your wishes. It
helps you see clearly into your own heart. One of the things
I have discovered there is that it's not what I do with my family that matters; it's doing it with them.

35.

I WAS IN Idaho fishing with Tim when David Carey called. I
usually don't answer my phone in the boat, but David knew
I was on vacation, so when I saw the call was from him, I
suspected that it was important.

It was. He told me he was stepping down as president of
Hearst Magazines and wanted to let me know before the
news was made public. A search would begin right away to
choose his successor. I told him I understood, wished him
well, and thanked him for letting me know. After I hung up,
I said to Tim, "I just lost my job."

Given the direction in which the print magazine business
was headed, it was clear to me that Hearst would replace
Carey with someone with more experience in digital publishing. A short time later, the head of Hearst's digital pub-

lishing operation was named as Carey's successor, and my boss, Joanna, resigned.

A month later, I was summoned to a conference room on the forty-fourth floor of the Hearst Tower, a slick corporate aerie with movie-worthy views of midtown Manhattan, and informed my services were no longer required. My tenure had lasted exactly one year.

The woman who delivered the news was someone who knew about my illness. Just a few weeks earlier, she had told me that her mother had cancer, and I had shared my story with her. Now she could barely choke out what she had to say before rushing from the room and leaving me with a human resources representative to discuss the details of my "termination," as the corporate euphemism goes.

The woman in question was someone I liked. My guess is that her boss, the new president of the company, had sent her to do his dirty work. She did not seem to enjoy it.

The consensus opinion on why I was let go was that the new president wanted to purge the old management team and put his own team into place. Fair enough. That happens all the time.

An alternative theory is that he took advantage of the moment to fire a relatively expensive employee who had cancer and might become deadweight at a time when he, like everyone else running a magazine company, desperately needed to cut costs. I have no way of knowing if that's true; possibly, I'm being unfair or even paranoid. But when you're sick, you wonder.

A short time later, I told that story to an HR professional I know. Without more information, she said she had no way to tell what might have really happened. She also told me that being sick can actually work to a person's advantage, since companies want to show that they're compliant with laws prohibiting discrimination against people with disabilities. Not that it was relevant to my situation—I had already been fired—but that possibility didn't sit well with me. I don't ever want to lose anything based on my health status, but I don't want to gain anything, either. I definitely don't want to be the token cancer patient. Those of us living with chronic illnesses and other disabilities have better things to worry about than helping a corporation meet a hiring quota. Other than reasonable accommodations, if we need them, we just want to be treated like everyone else. In or out of the workplace, we welcome your sympathy. You can keep your pity.

Regardless, I was now out of work in a dying industry where thousands of people were being laid off every year. Would I ever find another job? If so, how long would that take? Didi was working at *Shape* magazine, which was no better off financially than any other publication. What if she lost her job? Would we be able to get open-market medical insurance? Could we afford it? Would Dr. Richardson, Dr. Jagannath, and Dr. Gruenstein, who had successfully shepherded me through my diseases for almost fifteen years, be out of my new network and prohibitively expensive? How would Didi, A.J., and Oscar feel about having a spouse and parent who was out of work? Would they feel anxious? Afraid? Ashamed?

When I'd said that I hoped my job at Hearst might be the last job I ever had, that wasn't what I had meant.

36.

DIDI, A.J., OSCAR, and I, along with twenty or so other members of our extended family, typically spend Thanksgiving in

Boston, either at my brother Andy's house or my sister Tina's apartment. That fall, we celebrated at Tina's, with the usual food and festivities—two turkeys with all of the trimmings, lots and lots of desserts, and a poem Tina writes every year that's equal parts year in review, expression of gratitude, and family lampoon. That night, the four of us slept at Andy's house. The next morning, we had homemade scones with Andy and his wife, Kim, then headed home.

Like many people who live in Manhattan, Didi and I don't own a car, so we rent one when we take driving trips. I usually drop her and the kids in front of our apartment building when we get home, then return the car to the rental outlet a few blocks away. I had just done that and was walking home when my phone rang. It was Dr. Gruenstein. I'd had my quarterly scans and blood tests done the previous week. Dr. Gruenstein had received the results a few days before Thanksgiving but had been kind enough not to share them until after the holiday. He was calling to tell me my cancer was back.

Two or three years is considered an excellent response to RVD therapy. My remission had lasted for more than seven. In the spirit of the season, I wish I could say I was thankful for that good fortune, and in part, I was. I was also devastated. With a recurring, incurable illness, you want to believe, even though you 100 percent, without question, absolutely know better, that somehow it won't come back.

It does.

37.

I WAS SICK again, unemployed, and no longer seeing a therapist, so naturally, I went fishing. For my destination, I chose Chilean Patagonia, about as far away from New York as I could get. I lined up a story assignment, found a lodge, and headed south.

Patagonia is one of the world's most storied fly-fishing destinations, a place any angler worth their waders dreams of visiting. Fly-fishing enthusiasts can ply all manner of waters in the region, from big, rushing rivers to deep azure lakes to tiny, meandering creeks, and those waters hold fish in numbers and sizes that are hard to find anywhere else. Owing to the size of the area and the relative difficulty of getting there, much of it is still remarkably undeveloped. Even in the jet age, it is possible to find yourself fishing utterly alone, with no sign of civilization in sight. Comparisons to the American West of fifty or a hundred years ago are not inapt. I was there in December, at the start of the South American summer, in the Aysen region, near the city of Coyhaique, Chile.

The hour-long drive from the airport to the lodge was like an episode of *Nature*. The Andes loom in the distance, their summits dolloped with snow, and impossibly clear rivers wind through valleys that stretch to the horizon in every direction. You could spend a lifetime just naming the shades of green. On the dirt road that leads to the lodge, we got stuck for a time behind a herd of cattle being driven to pasture by gauchos. "Patagonian traffic jam," our shuttle driver said.

Guests are welcome to fish the lake next to the lodge as soon as they arrive, but because it was raining and cold on the afternoon I checked in, I enjoyed a pisco sour in front of the fireplace and chatted with the owner, Eduardo, about where we would fish during the week ahead. The son of a local schoolteacher, Eduardo is a born-and-bred resident of the area and lifelong fly-fisherman who knows every inch of the surrounding waters. With the help of a business partner and investor, Eduardo had built the lodge he and his wife,

Consuelo, now own and manage. The two of them are warm and gracious hosts: Eduardo manages the fishing operation, and Consuelo oversees the dining and lodging.

Dinner that night was an *asado*, or traditional Chilean barbecue, washed down with Chilean cabernet sauvignon and topped off with *leche nevada*, essentially a Chilean "floating island." By 10:00 P.M., I was in a deep asado-induced sleep.

The next morning, Eduardo and I drove to the Huemules River, named after a species of local deer that symbolizes Chileans' love of the outdoors and is featured on the country's national shield. We waded into the river at a spot just below a small, postcard-perfect waterfall that made for a memorable introduction to the watershed. Within half an hour of working our way upstream, I had caught and released my first Patagonian fish, a healthy, eighteen-inch brown trout. Unlike North American browns, that specimen had a distinctive spearmint color perfectly suited to its surroundings. The adaptation was uncanny, a Darwinian magic trick.

We went on to catch perhaps twenty more fish that day, rarely going longer than half an hour without a strike, and over the next four days, I fished every conceivable kind of water with remarkably consistent results. On day two, I fished the Simpson River, landing a particularly pretty twenty-inch rainbow. On day three, Eduardo and I fished Elizalde Lake. On my second cast, I caught a twenty-inch rainbow; minutes later, Eduardo one-upped me with a twenty-two-inch brown. (Guides don't always fish, but I was tired and encouraged him to have a go.) On day four, on another section of the Simpson River, we found a group of rainbows in a hole beneath an elevated bank. We landed five of them in fifteen minutes.

Day five was an especially memorable outing in which a

group of us—myself, two other guests, our guides, and a gaucho named Alfredo, whose family property abuts a section of the Mogotes River—rode horses to a stretch of that waterway. Fording the river on our mounts and clip-clopping along a narrow trail on the edge of a forty-foot cliff was an adventure in its own right. Lunch that day was a riverside picnic consisting of a whole, locally raised lamb roasted on a hand-carved spit over an open fire that Alfredo had prepared for the group. We washed it down with cans of ice-cold Escudo beer, a popular Chilean lager, that had been chilled in the river. It was like life imitating a beer commercial. If I had ever been in a flow state, I was in one then.

On the final morning of the trip, I found my white whale. My guides, Monte Becker and Hayden Dale, and I were on the Paloma River. We had begun the day by navigating a series of Class III rapids, then catching a handful of brown trout and rainbow trout that would have been considered whoppers on most other rivers, but here were just more in a series of ho-hum catches measuring eighteen inches or bigger.

Just before lunchtime, we ran a stretch of white water that squeezed between a pair of enormous boulders, then opened into a small, hidden canyon. With its overhanging granite walls, moody light, and silty water the color of sapphires (if the sapphires had somehow been electrified), the chamber bore traces of both the real-life Blue Lagoon and the fictional Middle-earth. It was one of the most striking spots I've seen, on or off a river.

For a time, we lingered there to fish, but with no luck. Then Monte rowed us downstream a few hundred feet to a small, unnamed island in the middle of the river, tied our inflatable raft to a tree stump, and instructed me to follow him to the top of a rock outcropping whose peak rose some thirty feet above the water. From that vantage point, we could see a near-perfect trout hideout: a clear, ice-blue pool protected on its upstream side by the island but still adjacent to the river's main current with its ready supply of insect life. He pointed to the head of a pool where he knew several sizable catches often lay. "Good fish," he said. "Rainbow."

Sure enough, there was a large, dark slab rising and falling in the water column, rhythmically picking flies off the surface for its lunch. We put him at just under twenty inches. A moment later, Monte said, "Look at the bottom of the pool. There's another one there. A big brown."

I scanned the area, but all I saw was an underwater log. Then the "log" rose to the surface and ate a fly. The object in question was, in fact, the largest trout I have ever seen outside Instagram, easily two feet long, possibly longer. He was exactly the sort of leviathan I had come to Patagonia for. Now all I had to do was catch him.

"Go ahead," Monte said. "Cast."

My first shot fell short, the second too far to the left. But my third attempt was on target, and I watched as my fly floated toward its mark.

The next thing I saw was a gaping mouth break the surface, then snap shut on my fly. I lifted my rod, and I'll be damned if I didn't hook him.

Although I didn't know it at the time, Hayden was filming the action on his phone. On the video, you can hear Monte say, "Nice brown!" then scramble down the rock toward the water to net my catch. My rod is bent nearly in half.

"I can't see him under the rock," I say to Monte. "Tell me if he—"

The fish briefly surfaces, no more than four feet from the net. Then my rod suddenly straightens, and I utter more than one of the seven words you can't say on television.

The fish is gone.

I have watched that video over and over, deconstructing it as though it were the Zapruder film. Maybe I should have put more pressure on the fish. Or less. Maybe I should have raised my rod tip more. Or lowered it. Maybe I should have hopped up and down on my left foot and declaimed "The Love Song of J. Alfred Prufrock." I'll never know.

We ate lunch on the rock, where I tried to be positive. Despite losing that brown, I told myself, I had just spent a week enjoying some of the best fishing, meals, wine, and company of my life. Still, I was miserable. Cancer can put a lot of things into perspective, but apparently, bringing the fish of a lifetime to within spitting distance of your net but then losing him isn't one of them.

After we finished eating, Monte and I walked back to the edge of the rock and looked down at the river. The rainbow, the first of the two fish we had seen there, was back in his spot. I caught him with one cast, then released him. I felt much better.

That night back at the lodge, as I was replaying the events of the day in my head, the phrase "It's always darkest before the dawn" came to mind. When I got home, I was scheduled to fly to Boston to talk to Dr. Richardson about what to do next. I could only hope that that hoariest of clichés was true.

PART SIX

Clinical Trial

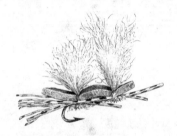

1.

I MET WITH Dr. Richardson in early January. We reviewed my symptoms and test results, and then, in his signature sunny way, he told me he had a "great new option" for me to consider. If I chose to, I could enroll in a clinical trial he was leading at Dana-Farber, in conjunction with other doctors and hospitals around the country: a pills-only protocol that I could take as an outpatient.

We tend to think of clinical trials as testing grounds for revolutionary lifesaving therapies that have not yet cleared the regulatory hurdles required to bring them to market. That is true in many instances, but trials also serve other purposes. Some investigate disease prevention measures. Others test diagnostic procedures. Others still weigh the effectiveness of combinations or dosages of drugs already approved and in use. At the time of this writing, there were more than a thousand clinical trials being conducted that focused on multiple myeloma alone, according to the Multiple Myeloma Research Foundation, a number that reflects the range of purposes for which clinical trials can be used.

Clinical trials occur in four phases. Phases I and II test the safety, efficacy, and side effects of a treatment on small (fifteen to thirty), then slightly larger (twenty-five to one hundred) numbers of people. In phase III trials, researchers compare the new treatment to the existing standard to be sure the new treatment is superior. Phase III trials involve from one hundred to several thousand people, with participants randomly assigned to one or the other of the treatments. Phase IV trials take place after a drug is approved by the FDA. Their purpose is to study the safety and efficacy of the treatment in the general population over the long term.

The trial Dr. Richardson wanted to enroll me in was a phase II trial involving two existing drugs called Pomalyst (generic name pomalidomide) and Ninlaro (generic name ixazomib)—new, souped-up, less toxic versions of Revlimid and Velcade that had been developed by Celgene and Takeda and initially approved in 2013 and 2015, respectively. Researchers frequently iterate on successful drugs to improve their safety and efficacy, and because I had done well on Revlimid and Velcade, it made sense for me to try their more advanced cousins. Pomalyst had become a new standard of care for relapsed myeloma patients (Dr. Richardson helped develop that drug, as well), and the purpose of the trial was to see if administering Ninlaro in combination with Pomalyst produced an added benefit.

Just three weeks earlier, I had been fording a river on horseback in Patagonia. Now I was sitting in my oncologist's office signing the release forms for an experimental cancer treatment.

2.

PATIENTS IN THE study I was participating in were divided into two groups, one that received only the Pomalyst and one that received both Pomalyst and Ninlaro. If one group showed significantly better results, the patients in the other would be switched to the more effective regimen.

I was randomly assigned to the Pomalyst-only group. The drug is taken daily in pill form, three weeks out of four, and I was to stay on it indefinitely. According to the study's guidelines, I was also required to take my old friend dexamethasone again, this time once a week. Because of the problems that drug had caused for me in the past, I asked if I could skip it or at least substitute something else, but under the trial's strict rules, that wasn't possible. What's more, the dex had to be taken in pill form, not intravenously, which tends to make its side effects more intense. In the past, I had seen Dr. Richardson once every three to six months, depending on how I was doing. To participate in the trial, I would have to travel to Boston once a month to have blood work and other tests done at Dana-Farber.

When I told one of Dr. Richardson's nurses about the problems I had had with dex, she suggested that I take the drug right before bed. That way, I could fall asleep before its effects kicked in, and its repercussions would be waning somewhat by the time I went to bed the following night.

I put the dex on the nightstand next to my bed, where I could take it, then immediately turned out the lights, but the strategy didn't work. I started the drug at 40 milligrams, the standard dosage, but had to be brought down to 30 milligrams, then 20, then 10, then 8, the lowest level the administrators of the trial would allow. Even at the 8-milligram dosage, I was more hyperactive and anxious on the oral dex than I had been on the IV form of the drug. I had more trouble sleeping (I was unable to do so for more than an hour or two for several nights after taking the medication), and my heartburn and hiccups returned. (On the plus side, I had the fullest beard I've ever had.) The dex also made my voice weak and reedy (it can thicken the tissues of your vocal cords), and because of the diaphragm issues the drug can cause, I had difficulty not just with hiccuping but also with breathing, especially whenever I bent over to, say, tie my shoes.

The dex also affected my poker game. At the time, we played on Monday night and I took the dex on Sundays.

Poker is, in large part, a game of judgment, and the drug impaired mine. I made overly aggressive decisions, and even when I tried to remind myself to play more cautiously, I would forget and play recklessly. It was like being drunk and trying to act sober. I had never been the best player at the table, but now I was consistently the worst. Thanks to the dex, losing also left me angry and depressed in a way it never had before. Things got so bad that I quit for a time. I returned a few months later, though. How else could I contribute to my friends' kids' college funds?

3.

A.J. WAS A sophomore in high school. To pursue her love of singing and acting, she had applied to the Fiorello H. LaGuardia High School of Music & Art and Performing Arts and been accepted into its voice program. She also joined a weekend theater group and attended a performing arts summer camp during those years, playing Audrey in *Little Shop of Horrors*, Patrice in *13*, Jenny in *Company*, and Beth in *Merrily We Roll Along*, and she sang in her high school choir. That year, she came out as queer and had her first serious girlfriend.

Oscar, meanwhile, was in middle school and had become interested in what's called circus arts. He attended the same summer camp as A.J., and one of the activities on offer was a Cirque du Soleil–style program, with tumbling, rope climbing, and flying trapeze. Oscar, who has always had both an artsy and an athletic side, was taken by it. After he came home that summer, Didi found him a circus school in the city that he wound up attending for several years. Oz, as we sometimes call him, was also into piano (Didi's mother was thrilled), tennis, and restaurants and cooking. He and I began eating our way through the many cuisines on offer in New York and preparing sometimes elaborate dinners together at home.

Shortly after I met with Dr. Richardson to determine my new treatment plan, A.J. suffered a medical emergency. While Didi and I were in the ER waiting for the doctors' assessment, my cellphone rang. It was a patient coordinator from Dr. Richardson's office calling to speak to me about my first clinical trial appointment later that week.

As humans, we like to imagine that if one awful thing is happening, a second one can't happen at the same time. But the universe has no such fairness clause. There is no upper limit on the number of problems you can have at once. Your daughter can be in the hospital at the very moment an oncology nurse calls to discuss your impending experimental cancer treatment.

After I hung up, I went numb. Mercifully, A.J.'s emergency passed, but at that moment, I felt overwhelmed. It was as close as I had come since my diagnosis to feeling hopeless. It was as close as I had come to thinking, *I can't do this.*

4.

FOR MY MONTHLY checkups in Boston, I had to do a twenty-four-hour urine test and take the sample along with me. Because post-9/11 FAA rules prohibit passengers from carrying liquids of 3.5 ounces or more per container onto a plane, carrying a half-gallon jug of urine with me presented a problem. I could have driven to Boston or taken a train or bus, but those modes of transportation took significantly longer than flying, and whenever I went to Dr. Richardson's, I liked to get the visit over with as quickly as possible and return home to my regular life.

Dr. Richardson provided me with a letter explaining my situation, and when I got to the Delta security checkpoint at LaGuardia Airport on my way to my first appointment, I told the TSA agent what I was carrying and why and showed him the note. I'm not sure if he was skeptical or just extremely dutiful, but he proceeded to unscrew the cap of the bottle and . . . sniff it. Next, he dipped a piece of litmus paper into the jug and waited a few seconds for the result. Then he looked at me and nodded for me to be on my way. He was a model of professionalism. I hope he got hazard pay.

My first checkup with Dr. Richardson went fine. My brother, Andy, came to the appointment, too, and we had our usual weird but lovely visit. It was too soon to tell if the Pomalyst was working, but my physical exam, my vital signs, and my basic blood tests were all good. I answered a series of standard questions required by the clinical trial protocol, filled out a handful of forms, left my jug full of urine with a nurse, and turned around and flew home.

5.

LATER THAT MONTH, I was brushing my teeth one morning when I felt something strange on the outside wall of my gums, above my top left wisdom tooth. It wasn't a lump or bump; it was more like a hole—an absence, not a presence.

It turned out to be osteonecrosis of the jaw. When a portion of the jawbone dies, it can cause the gum tissue to pull away from the affected spot. The condition was clearly caused by the Zometa (by that time, I'd had upward of a hundred doses), by the switch I had made to Xgeva, or both.

Doctors don't understand why those medications sometimes trigger ONJ, and the severity of the condition varies wildly, with some patients losing only a small chip of bone and others losing part or all of their jaw. There are no effective treatments; intervening often makes the problem worse.

I got lucky. After several months of being followed by a dental oncologist, yet another subspecialty I hadn't previously known existed, a small piece of my jawbone chipped off, the hole in my gum returned to normal, and the condition didn't spread.

At my next clinical trial checkup, Dr. Richardson switched me to a bone strengthener called Aredia (generic name pamidronate disodium) that's less likely to cause ONJ but takes two hours to administer, more than twice as long as Zometa and far longer than an Xgeva shot. I was fine with the trade-off.

6.

ON THE JOB search front, it was time to get out of print magazine publishing. As much as I enjoyed what I did, the industry's decline was accelerating; every day seemed to bring news of publications laying people off or closing. I didn't want to get onto that train to nowhere again.

Among traditional magazines, *New York* got into the digital publishing game relatively early. Although I didn't work directly on its website, I did do some overlapping work and was exposed to how it operated. There and at *Vogue,* I had picked up just enough experience to be a credible candidate for digital publishing jobs. That side of the business, although still nascent and destined to be beset by its own economic challenges, was at least oriented toward the future. I concentrated my job search there.

A friend of Didi's is married to someone who worked at Medium, the online publishing platform founded by Evan Williams, one of Twitter's cofounders. He was kind enough to introduce me to Ev; Ev, in turn, introduced me to Medium's head of editorial, Siobhan O'Connor, and after several rounds of interviews, I wound up getting a job offer. I started on March 1, 2019.

Medium's strategy at the time was to launch a group of digital publications. My job was to help Siobhan do that. It was an incredible opportunity. Essentially, I got to recruit and hire dozens of talented writers and editors and help them invent publications covering politics, race, technology, business, health, and more. We had budgets like most of us hadn't seen in years, and our mandate, issued by Ev, was to produce "world-class journalism." It was as though someone had turned back the clock to the good old days of the magazine business.

One night, a few months after I started, the editor of one of the new publications and I were working late. He had been at the company for only a few weeks and was still dumbstruck by his good fortune. "I just hope," he said, "this lasts."

7.

IN OCTOBER 2019, I visited my father at a hospice facility near his home in Massachusetts. A little more than a year earlier, he had been taking a walk when he had found himself dizzy and out of breath. He had called my mother, who took him to the hospital. After a series of tests and doctors appointments, he had been diagnosed with a failing heart valve. He had the valve replaced that fall, and while the surgery had been nominally successful, he was never quite the same. He tired easily. He sometimes struggled to conjure a memory or thought. His speech was occasionally slurred.

The following July, we threw a party for his ninetieth birthday. All four of his children and most of his nine grandchildren were there, plus their spouses and significant others. My father's brother, Milton, was there, as was his sister, Rena, who'd flown in from her home in Tel Aviv. After dinner, everyone shared their favorite memory of "Pop." The details varied, but the themes were the same: The man would show up for you. He loved to tell a good joke. He was uncommonly kind.

And then my father spoke. First, he recounted his career—the Amsterdam Printing Company, *Wilderness Camping,* his own consulting business. His point wasn't to call attention to his accomplishments; it was to express wonder that a child of immigrant parents who had come off the boat without money or formal education or knowing the language of their new home had somehow managed to successfully build a career and raise a family. He seemed awed by the thought of it, as if he had witnessed a miracle.

He expressed his love for my mother and noted that they had been married for sixty-two years. He looked at her and repeated the phrase for emphasis: "*Sixty-two years.*" He finished by saying that he'd had a good life, that he was grateful for it, and that he owed it to all of us.

There were a lot of soggy "Happy 90th!" napkins.

The end of my father's life was no less awful for following a familiar arc. He began having frequent dizzy spells, sometimes falling and winding up in the emergency room. He was in and out of hospitals and rehabilitation facilities. There were procedures and medications, plus medications to treat complications of the procedures. Because his decline took place over several months, many of his family and friends got to spend time with him before he died.

In the hospice facility, my father was frail and weak. His skin was pale and paper thin. He had stopped eating and was experiencing hallucinations from the morphine he was being given to manage his pain. At one point, he told me to look out the window; he saw a zeppelin drifting by. We talked about the news of the day and watched the New England Patriots play on TV. (After years of living in Massachusetts, my father had converted from a New York Giants fan to a Patriots fan. I said he was a wonderful man; I did not say he was perfect.) He asked about my family and job. Then, he asked if I had any fishing trips planned.

He often asked me that. Over the years, we had established a routine where I would text him pictures of fish I had caught and later tell him the story behind them. At various points, I had sent him shots of bonefish I had landed in the Bahamas, redfish in Texas, striped bass off Montauk, rainbow trout in Montana, brook trout in the Great Smoky Mountains. I told him I was planning to go to Idaho soon to fish. He seemed to take in that information, but then his mind appeared to wander. He saw another zeppelin.

Then, his thinking appeared to clear. "Remember the day we fished together?" he asked. He paused. Every sentence was an effort. "That was fun."

He died peacefully a week later. Amid my grief, I was relieved: He had never had to bury a child. To this day, I text him pictures of the notable fish I catch. I know he doesn't get them, but I send them anyway.

Before my father died, he asked that in lieu of flowers to honor his memory, donations be made to the Multiple Myeloma Research Foundation. I can't think of anything that better captures who he was.

8.

FOR SOME THIRTY years, my parents had been snowbirds. They had spent summers in Massachusetts and winters in Florida. After my father died, my mother decided to go to Florida as she normally would. My siblings and I had encouraged her to stay north, closer to us, but she wanted to stick to her routine. At age eighty-eight, she was still remarkably healthy, physically speaking. She still walked and swam every day. The trouble was that she had been suffering from dementia for a number of years—she'd had episodes of severe memory loss and was no longer capable of driving—and it was my father who had kept her safe and functioning. Now she would be living on her own. My sisters arranged for caregivers to go to her house daily to check on her, keep her company, and take her shopping, and we crossed our fingers.

One day that December, my mother fainted and fell. The home healthcare aide who was with her took her to the hospital and was kind enough to visit her there several times until one of us could fly to Florida. Andy, who lives half an hour from what was then my parents' Massachusetts home, had been the primary caregiver to my father when he was dying, and Jen and Tina had done the lion's share of the work involved in taking care of my mother since my father had passed away. It was my turn to pitch in, if only in a small way. I flew to Florida.

My mother had been discharged from the hospital and was home (her doctor said her fall had been caused by exhaustion and dehydration related to grieving). She looked sad and somewhat frail but remarkably vital for someone who had just lost her husband and then been hospitalized for two days.

That afternoon, my mother and I sat on her patio and talked. She asked about me, Didi, and the kids, and in turn, I asked how she was doing.

She was tired, she said, and lonesome. Adjusting to living on her own was more difficult than she had expected. There was a lot of downtime to fill, and many of the couples she and my father used to have dinner or go to the movies with were not interested in socializing with a single person. When she said she missed my father and was grateful for the time they'd had together, she choked up. We exchanged some happy memories of him, and that seemed to cheer her up.

Then she began to fade. It had been years since she had asked me about my illness, and she seemed to have no awareness of it. Dementia is an awful disease that takes a tremendous toll on those who suffer from it and on their loved ones. By no means should the havoc it can wreak be underestimated. At the same time, I couldn't help but wonder as I sat there with my mother: Could forgetting the painful parts of your life, at least in some sense, be a good thing?

9.

SHORTLY AFTER I got home from Florida, I was riding the stationary bike at my gym when I saw an ad on television encouraging people who believed they were eligible for the September 11th Victim Compensation Fund to file a claim.

The fund had been established on September 22, 2001, to aid people who were injured or killed as a result of the 9/11 terrorist attacks and the cleanup that had followed. Intended to help those most directly affected by the attacks, the original fund had been closed in 2004.

In 2010, Congress enacted the Zadroga Act, expanding the eligibility criteria for victims. In part, the measure was passed to include people who had been living or working in or near the World Trade Center during and after the attacks who had been diagnosed with cancer. The Zadroga Act was reauthorized in 2015 and permanently authorized in 2019. To date, more than $7 billion has been distributed to victims.

The administrators of the fund established a list of cancers linked to 9/11. Multiple myeloma is one of them. They also established a geographical zone of eligibility bordered on the north by Canal Street. At the time of the attacks, I lived thirteen blocks north of it, and I haven't lived more than sixteen blocks from Canal Street since. At that time and for the following year and a half, I had also worked seven blocks north of that dividing line.

I had seen the TV ads before, but for some reason, I was moved that morning to call the displayed telephone number. In the years since I had been diagnosed, I had become increasingly convinced that it was the toxic fallout from the World Trade Center attacks that had caused my illness. Nothing else I had learned in the intervening years about multiple myeloma suggested any other cause. It was Occam's razor: The simplest explanation is the likeliest one. Although I knew that the eligibility cutoff was Canal Street, I decided to see if exceptions were ever made.

The woman who answered the phone sounded like an intern or a paralegal. She asked me a handful of questions, including where I had lived and worked at the time. When I told her I had worked seven blocks north of Canal Street and asked if there was any flexibility on that front, she said that, unfortunately, there was not.

"Doesn't that seem arbitrary?" I said. "I lived so close to the cutoff line. The air couldn't have been much better there than it was below the line."

She said she understood, but a line had to be drawn somewhere. She was sorry, but there was nothing she could do. Life is sometimes a game of inches. Or blocks, anyway.

For a moment, I said nothing. I was angry, but I also knew she was right. A line did have to be drawn. I felt awkward making the call in the first place. Was I looking for a hand-out? Did I deserve compensation? What if it wasn't 9/11 that had made me sick? Besides, the woman I was speaking to had been nothing but kind. If anything, I had the sense that if she could have helped me, she would have.

I told her I understood and thanked her for her time.

"You're welcome," she said. "Good luck."

10.

IN FEBRUARY 2020, I took a business trip to San Francisco. Medium's headquarters was there, and the company was hosting a series of employee training sessions. During my three-day stay, I attended the meetings, had dinners with colleagues and friends, and revisited some of my old haunts. The day after I got home, I came down with a bug. I had a fever and chills and was so tired I could hardly get out of bed.

I never had the telltale cough typical of the first wave of the covid pandemic. I felt better in a matter of days, and I later tested negative for covid antibodies. But in retrospect, I was lucky that I didn't contract the disease. As the world now knows, the virus that causes covid had been circulating in the United States as early as December and was widespread by February. Flying across the country, passing through busy airports, sitting in cramped, poorly ventilated conference rooms all day, and eating in crowded restaurants, all as a cancer patient with compromised immunity, I was at high risk of contracting the illness. I felt as though I had dodged a viral bullet.

A few weeks later, Didi, A.J., Oscar, and I went into lock-down along with the rest of the country and most of the world. As one of the epicenters of the disease, New York was hit particularly hard. Hospitals were overrun, hundreds of people were dying every day, and temporary morgues were set up around the city. Every evening at seven, Didi, A.J., Oscar, and I stuck our heads out of our windows and cheered along with our neighbors in support of healthcare and other essential workers. It was a frightening and heartbreaking time to live in the city.

Although many people were moving out of New York, either temporarily or for good, Didi and I decided to stay. We don't own a second home, and we didn't feel right put-ting our family or friends at increased risk by adding peo-ple to their households. If we followed the recommended protocols—quarantining, social distancing, masking, test-ing as appropriate—we reasoned we'd be safe.

To pass the time in lockdown, we read books, streamed TV shows, and took walks along the Hudson River. A.J., who was a junior in high school, learned to crochet. Oscar, who was in sixth grade, taught himself how to bake bread. We went to the grocery store at off-hours, ordered pretty much everything else we needed online, and limited our so-cial contact to people in our "bubble."

With schools and businesses closed, we worked and went to school by Zoom. At roughly a thousand square feet, our apartment is small for four people. It's really a two-bedroom, but we converted the dining room into a third bedroom after Oscar was born. Several years earlier, A.J. had found a stray cat we had adopted and named Batman (as a kitten, he looked exactly like a bat). With four humans and two cats living under one roof, space was not something we had in excess.

At one point early in the lockdown, Didi set up her laptop

at our kitchen table for a Zoom meeting. I did the same thing in a reading chair in a corner of our bedroom. For the foreseeable future, those spaces became our home offices. As people who, more or less, type and have meetings for a living, Didi and I were fortunate: We could keep our jobs and work from home.

Didi hated it. She's extremely social. The more people she's around and the more often, the better. I didn't mind it. The advantages of working from home for someone who needs to avoid germs are obvious, and although I missed my colleagues, not going to an office every day taught me that I'm something of a closet introvert. I was never unhappy in social settings, and I'm still not. I like attending work meetings, having dinner out, and going to the movies as much as the next person. But I discovered I like being alone more than I'd thought I did. For me, solitude is at once calming and energizing. Working at home, I was able to control the balance between social me and private me more to my liking.

A.J. and Oscar hated Zoom school but slogged through it in their respective bedrooms. As the older of the two, A.J. mastered the art of skipping virtual classes by going "camera off" faster than her brother, but neither of them was above using the trick. As it was for so many kids, that semester of school was largely a waste.

As the lockdown was extended first for weeks, then for months, bars, restaurants, and shops in our neighborhood began to close; companies, including Medium, announced that they were permanently shuttering their brick-and-mortar offices; and more and more people moved out of the city. It occurred to me that a strange phenomenon was taking shape. It was the first time many healthy people were living in my world. Everyone was worried about getting sick. Everyone was facing uncertainty.

11.

FOR A TIME, the fact that I couldn't travel to Boston for my monthly checkups appeared to render me ineligible for the clinical trial. Fortunately, the study's administrators changed the rules and temporarily allowed Zoom appointments.

In May, during my regular video appointment, Dr. Richardson told me the clinical trial protocol wasn't working. Not well enough, anyway. I had no new bone lesions, but my most recent blood work showed my M protein level to be ticking up and certain markers of my immune system health to be abnormal. Dr. Richardson decided to add the second drug being studied in the trial, Ninlaro, to my regimen to see if that would help.

Unlike its predecessor, Velcade, which is administered by IV, Ninlaro could be taken in pill form. That was the good news. The bad news was that Ninlaro brought on a side effect I hadn't previously experienced: brain fog. I had trouble focusing. I was forgetful. I would start a sentence and lose track of where I was going before I could finish it. I hadn't contracted covid, but ironically enough, I was experiencing one of the telltale symptoms of long covid, the debilitating and poorly understood condition many covid patients had begun suffering from.

In June, when the administrators of the clinical trial revoked the Zoom meeting exception, I made my way to La-Guardia Airport. It was the first time I had flown, to Boston or anywhere else, since lockdown. The Delta terminal at La-Guardia during rush hour on a Monday morning is usually filled with people. That day, it was just me and the TSA agents. Literally. There was not a single other flier.

To make those trips to Boston, I wore not one but two KN-95 masks at all times (like most other people in the early days of the pandemic, I was unable to get the higher-quality

N-95 masks) and washed my hands and used hand sanitizer religiously. I stopped short of wearing a face shield. Some fates are worse than death.

I was still nervous about getting sick from traveling, but I had no real choice. If I wanted to stay in the clinical trial, which was clearly what Dr. Richardson thought was best for me and was serving me well, I had to go to Boston. Flying was perhaps less safe than driving, but I decided that the advantage in speed was worth it. I masked up, bought more Purell, and resumed my monthly trips.

12.

LATER THAT MONTH, I was supposed to go fishing in Alaska. I had been dreaming of doing so for years and had landed a magazine assignment to explore the waters of the Kenai Peninsula, a choice destination for king salmon and other species, but covid forced me to cancel the trip. Flying to Boston to receive cancer treatment was one thing; flying to Alaska to catch fish didn't seem wise.

Ever since I got sick, I've tried to be strategic about making plans. The closer I get to a retesting period, the fewer I make. That goes for everything from coffees with friends to fishing excursions. When PET scans and marrow biopsies are on the horizon, planning ahead seems too precarious. More than once I've disregarded that strategy, only to have to cancel everything on my calendar because I have new symptoms or need new treatment. Man plans, cancer laughs. That time, covid got in the way. Instead of jetting off to Alaska, I took the elevator from my apartment down to the lobby of my building and headed out to West Twelfth Street.

A number of years earlier, looking to shake off the rust and get my arm into shape for an upcoming fishing trip, I'd wanted to do some practice casting. But living where I do, I didn't have a suitable place to do so. Or I thought I didn't. Then it occurred to me that a city street—long, straight, and, in my case, relatively free of traffic—is actually quite suitable. Pretty great, even.

Early one Sunday morning, when there weren't too many cars around, I planted myself in front of my building and commenced slinging thirty or forty feet of thin nylon line behind me and in front of me, over and over again, while stepping into and out of the street in sync with the traffic light cycles to avoid passing cars. I called it street casting— essentially fly-fishing without the fish—and it was exactly as strange as it sounds.

With traveling to fish more or less off the table while covid raged, street casting took on a new urgency. I started indulging in the madness almost every day.

While street casting, per se, may not be an actual thing, fly casting definitely is. The sport dates back some 150 years and was popular enough in the first half of the twentieth century that competitions were held at Madison Square Garden. Today, the pursuit is centered mostly on local clubs, with various associations around the world hosting distance and accuracy competitions.

There's a simple pleasure in the metronomic rhythms of fly casting, and it's a pretty cool experiment in applied physics. The trick is to "load" the line on the back cast, then transfer the coiled energy on the forward cast, stopping the rod at precisely the right moment to shoot the line forward with maximum speed. With so many variables in play, a million things can go wrong. But when you get it right, it's magic.

In some ways, casting in the street isn't all that different from casting on a river. For safety reasons, I cut the hook off the fly, and I practice my accuracy by aiming for things such as street signs and manholes. They're not exactly rising trout, but they do. Any distance constraints the street presents aren't really an issue, at least not for me. Championship casters regularly shoot line well over two hundred feet—the current U.S. record stands at an astonishing 243 feet—but I'm more of a thirty-foot guy.

The casting itself is only part of the attraction. It's also fun just to do something weird. Just about everyone who passes by me on the sidewalk stops, gawks, or comments. Roughly half of them ask, "Catch anything?" The more self-conscious among them note that I probably get that all the time. For the record, that does not make the question any less awkward.

At the same time, a certain kind of blithe New Yorker will affect a "no big deal" attitude when they see me, as if the strange tableau they've come upon is something they've beheld a thousand times before. One Sunday morning, a woman who looked to be at least ninety walked past me on the sidewalk without so much as slowing down. "I've lived in this neighborhood my whole life," she said, as much to the universe as to me or anyone else. "*That* I have never seen."

13.

IN OCTOBER 2020, I was scheduled to give a company-wide virtual presentation one day at work, but the brain fog the Ninlaro was causing made the prospect daunting. I spoke to Siobhan and told her I wasn't sure I could do it. She knew about my illness; earlier, I had explained to her why I was traveling to Boston once a month.

You might not think the inability to give a run-of-the-mill Tuesday afternoon PowerPoint presentation would be that big a deal, but it threw me. It was the first time I wasn't able to perform a work task because of my illness. Was it a step toward disability? Toward losing my job? My insurance? If I couldn't be professional me, how would I help support my family? Who would I be? Also, brain fog is frightening. You wonder if you might be losing your mind.

On a simpler level, I felt guilty about not being able to give the presentation. But Siobhan understood. She confided in me that she had lost her brother, who she told me had also been her best friend, to cancer. She gave the presentation for me.

14.

A FEW WEEKS later, I put on a pair of sunglasses to go out for a walk and felt something odd on the bridge of my nose. I remembered having been hit by a wave while bodysurfing the previous summer and that my sunglasses had hit that spot. Maybe I had damaged the bone. Then, I ran my finger over the area and felt a bump underneath the skin. A bone biopsy determined that it was a myeloma lesion. I wound up having another round of radiation, fifteen sessions between Thanksgiving and Christmas, midpandemic, Lecter Mask included.

On average, the clinical trial I was on found that Pomalyst and Ninlaro effectively controlled multiple myeloma for two years. For me, the drugs had worked for roughly a year and a half. It's possible I may have had a better response if I had been on both drugs from the start, but that was a risk of the trial. On the plus side, my response was good: The trial kept my disease well controlled for a significant period of time. In any case, there was no going back. It was time to move on.

PART SEVEN

Immunotherapy

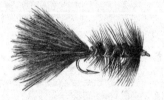

1.

THERE I WAS, in Dr. Richardson's office again. And there he was, outlining another treatment plan for me. He told me he wanted to move me off the Pomalyst and Ninlaro and on to another two-drug cocktail made up of medications called Darzalex (generic name daratumumab) and Kyprolis (generic name carfilzomib), two more weapons in the fight against myeloma that had been developed in, incredibly enough, the years since I had been diagnosed.

Developed by Janssen Pharmaceutical Companies and approved for use in multiple myeloma in 2015, Darzalex was one of the first monoclonal antibodies approved for myeloma. Variously described as a targeted therapy and an immunotherapy, it works by binding to a protein called CD38 that is overexpressed on myeloma cells, then inducing the death of those cells through multiple mechanisms. Developed by doctors at Yale University and the biotech company Proteolix, and approved for use in multiple myeloma in 2012, Kyprolis is a next-generation proteasome inhibitor similar to Velcade and Ninlaro.

The two drugs would be administered by IV infusion once a week for six months, along with dexamethasone. Because I was no longer involved in the Dana-Farber clinical trial, I could get my treatments at home in New York, at Dr. Gruenstein's office. (Somewhere, a TSA agent was smiling.)

I started my immunotherapy infusions in January 2021, scheduling them for Monday mornings, first thing. My intention was to get my treatment over with as quickly as possible, then get on with the rest of my week.

Since the time I had gotten my RVD treatments there, Dr.

Gruenstein's practice had been purchased by a large cancer care conglomerate, and the treatment room at his office was now a much bigger, busier space. Instead of five or six oncological BarcaLoungers, there were now twenty-five or thirty. Because of the pandemic, patients and staff were required to wear masks, and the staff was scrupulous about wearing gloves and disinfecting the chairs, IV poles, and other equipment after each use. The fact that the doctors and nurses were risking their own safety for the sake of their patients wasn't lost on me. The work they and other healthcare and frontline workers did during the pandemic was heroic.

About ten minutes into my first treatment session, a nurse checked on me and noticed a rash on my face. She asked to look at my chest and discovered red blotches there, too. She summoned Dr. Gruenstein, who said I was having an allergic reaction and switched my IV drip from the immunotherapy medicines to Benadryl. It was like the first day of my RVD treatment all over again, oncological déjà vu. The rash disappeared, and I fell into a Benadryl-induced sleep.

The Darzalex and Kyprolis didn't bother me much. Although Kyprolis can sometimes cause serious heart and lung problems, I experienced neither of those issues. Yet again, I didn't lose my hair (neither Darzalex nor Kyprolis commonly causes hair loss), and the brain fog I had experienced from the Ninlaro disappeared.

The dex, however, was still a burden. I slept for maybe two hours on Monday nights and three or four on Tuesdays before getting back to my normal sleep pattern. It felt like extreme jet lag, like I was flying to Tokyo once a week.

As much as anything, the new treatment regimen was a grind. It took more than four hours to administer, twice as long as the RVD therapy had required, and a cumulative fatigue began to set in, not just from the weekly infusions but from all of the previous treatments I'd had over the years.

I'm generally a punctual person, but I started showing up late for my infusion appointments, sometimes very late. It was as if my mind knew when I was supposed to leave my apartment, but my arms and legs wouldn't cooperate. The body knows where it does and doesn't want to go.

A few weeks into my treatment, I realized that I had been wearing the same outfit to every appointment: a North Face fleece, Adidas sweatpants, and a T-shirt with the Medium logo on it, all black. Not that I had done it purposely, but it occurred to me later that the color selection had reflected my mood.

Before the pandemic, I would have considered opting for a cab over the subway as sacrilege. Riding the subway (and complaining about it) is one of the things that makes a New Yorker a New Yorker. But like many people at that time, I sought to avoid the germs of the underground as much as possible. Instead, I took taxis or Ubers to and from my appointments each week.

Every Monday morning, I would ride up to Dr. Gruenstein's office on Madison Avenue and Eighty-sixth Street, past the expensive shops and boutiques, get my treatment, then ride home down Fifth Avenue, past Central Park, St. Patrick's Cathedral, Rockefeller Center, the New York Public Library, and the Empire State Building.

The trips had a cognitive dissonance about them. It was as though I were a tourist on one of those double-decker sight-seeing buses, except that I wasn't taking the rides to see the sights; I was taking them because I was sick. I was cancer commuting.

2.

IN MARCH 2021, a few days after I got my first covid vaccination, I mentioned to the nurse who was giving me my Darzalex infusion that I was feeling a little less worried about getting the disease. There was an awkward pause. Actually, he said, I might not be protected. For people who are immunocompromised, he told me, vaccines aren't always effective. If your body's immune system isn't at full strength, you're not able to produce the antibodies a vaccine is meant to stimulate. As a result, you may or may not develop a sufficient level of antibodies to fight off or even minimize the effects of the illness the shot is meant to guard against. In my case, both my myeloma and the treatment I'd received had damaged my immune system. The only way to find out if I had developed an effective level of covid antibodies was to be tested.

In May, I had that test done; it's a simple blood test. I had developed a small number of antibodies but not nearly enough to keep me safe from a covid infection.

In July, I got a third covid shot, and in August, I got retested. I had more antibodies, but still not enough.

In September, I got shot number four. That one finally did the trick.

With each new shot since—each shot developed for each new variant, that is—I've had to do similar repeats.

3.

IN APRIL, FOUR months into my Darzalex and Kyprolis treatments, I was shaving one morning when I noticed a rough, dry patch of red skin on my forehead. I made an appointment with my dermatologist. One biopsy and a week or so later, she called to say that I had skin cancer. When I asked her if the condition might be related to myeloma, she explained that being immunocompromised doesn't just leave you more susceptible to infectious diseases, it leaves you more vulnerable to all illnesses. Cancer begets cancer.

Fortunately, the malignancy was squamous cell cancer, not one of the more dangerous forms, but I still needed surgery to remove it to make sure it didn't spread. It is a twisted fact of being a myeloma patient that less aggressive cancers seem acceptable by comparison.

In June, I learned that a key measure of my immune system health called immunoglobulin G, or IgG, had dropped to dangerously low levels. (Because the regimen I was on frequently causes IgG decreases, I was being tested regularly for that issue.) Antibodies by a different name, immunoglobulins are the proteins produced by plasma cells to kill viruses, bacteria, and other germs when your body senses that it's under attack. IgG is the most common of the five immunoglobulins (the others are immunoglobulin A, M, D, and E) and is critical for fighting infections. Because of my deficiency, I had to add a monthly dose of intravenous IgG, or IVIG for short, to my treatment regimen. That infusion took up to six hours to administer. On one out of every four trips to Dr. Gruenstein's treatment room, my treatments were now that much longer. I also had to cancel my Alaska fly-fishing trip and magazine assignment for the second summer in a row. Until I could get my IgG levels up, Dr. Gruenstein said, it wasn't smart for me to travel.

4.

AT MEDIUM, THE new publications we started were producing widely read and well-received stories. Because the pandemic created an enormous appetite for health information, our health publication, *Elemental,* was doing particularly well. But the new entities were also expensive to run, and the company's growth had slowed. Medium is a subscription-only business—it doesn't accept advertising—and after a pandemic-induced spike, the number of new subscribers was trailing off. Rumors began circulating that management was losing faith in the new publications.

In 2018, Didi had moved out of publishing and into a hybrid of journalism and advertising called content marketing. She worked on travel, finance, and other accounts for an agency that was well established and stable. Her job seemed secure. But we still didn't feel comfortable unless we had a two-tiered employment situation. And for me, the specter of the Great Media Die-off was once again looming.

5.

ON THE MORNING of June 23, 2021, Didi and I took an Uber to Central Park. Because of the pandemic, A.J.'s high school graduation was being held there instead of in her school's auditorium.

It was a Kodachrome summer morning, all buttery yellows, royal blues, and kelly greens. The keynote speaker talked about covid, the unprecedented challenges the class of 2021 had faced, and the adaptability and resilience they had displayed. "Pomp and Circumstance" was played, the diplomas were handed out, and the kids tossed their caps. After all of the disruptions of the previous year, the familiar rituals felt comforting.

Afterward, Didi, Oscar, and I joined A.J. and a group of her friends and their families for lunch at a restaurant. We were seated indoors, in a large, well-ventilated space that felt reasonably safe. I wouldn't have missed it, regardless.

Do you remember how, shortly after my diagnosis, I had asked God to let me live to see A.J.'s high school graduation? For anyone seeking proof of prayers being answered, this would be a compelling piece of evidence.

The following month, after I completed the six months of Darzalex and Kyprolis therapy Dr. Richardson had prescribed, I saw him in Boston for a checkup. Based on my most recent blood tests, he told me, the treatment had worked partially, but it hadn't produced a complete response. I would have to continue the regimen for another three months and increase the Kyprolis dosage. The Monday-morning fun at Dr. Gruenstein's office would continue.

6 .

THAT FALL, A.J. started college. Because she had been a junior in high school when the pandemic had begun, she hadn't been able to tour prospective schools. They weren't allowing it. But she knew she wanted to attend a small liberal arts college and to get out of New York. She was tired of city living, especially amid the pandemic. A friend from her weekend theater group whom she liked and admired was attending Kenyon College in Gambier, Ohio. A.J. applied early and was accepted.

In August, Didi and I rented a car, packed it up with A.J.'s things, and drove her to school (with brief exceptions, Kenyon held in-person classes throughout the pandemic). Didi and I both felt the same way about our oldest child heading off to college: We would miss her terribly, of course, but we were thrilled she was starting such an exciting new part of her life. For me, it was also another milestone. I had been so focused on making it to her high school graduation that I had forgotten about her starting college. That didn't make it any less wonderful.

7.

THE UNWELCOME MEDICAL news kept coming.

In September, I woke up one morning with blurred vision and "floaters" in both eyes. This turned out to be something called posterior vitreous detachment, or PVD, in which bits of the gellike substance called vitreous humor that fills the space between the lens and the retina in the human eye break loose. Fortunately, the condition went away on its own in a matter of months as the bits broke down into smaller and smaller pieces. Better still, I wasn't having a stroke. My ophthalmologist told me that PVD is often caused by steroids such as dexamethasone.

Then, in November, I was diagnosed with a benign enlarged prostate. At least, that was a perfectly common medical condition. I viewed it as a prize for reaching middle age.

8.

EARLY IN 2022, with covid infections rapidly falling, many people had begun to believe that the pandemic was over and had stopped getting vaccinated, wearing masks, and taking other precautions. That posed a problem for me and the millions of other immunocompromised people around the world. That January, I wrote an op-ed essay for *The Washington Post* called "This Is a Dangerous Time in the Pandemic for People Like Me. Don't Forget Us." In it I urged readers to consider the needs of cancer patients and others who are immunocompromised as they moved forward.

"I understand why anyone who is healthy, or better still, healthy and vaccinated, would be eager to let down their guard," I wrote. "Early data suggest omicron is less likely than other variants to lead to hospitalizations and deaths, particularly in immunized people. And who wants to live with pandemic restrictions for one second longer than they have to?

"The problem with that calculus, though, is that it doesn't account for everyone. As more and more people decide to just live with the virus, or even try to deliberately contract it to 'get it over with,' the immunocompromised and other vulnerable populations are being forgotten."

The story touched a nerve. It was read by more than 150,000 people and generated some 1,300 comments. Many people offered supportive thoughts, such as "This far into this pandemic, we shouldn't have to be having this conversation. Pleading with others to yield to decency is becoming exhausting." And "Thank you for this beautiful essay— I hope it reminds everyone of how important it is to protect the most vulnerable."

Others shared less sympathetic points of view. "We are tired of people like you trying to dictate our lives . . . ," one reader wrote. "Live in fear as you wish. Fully vaccinated, boosted, healthy, not elderly, and a good weight, I am good with my risks."

"It's selfish of you to ask everyone else to sacrifice their mental health," another reader offered. "You should stay home."

Still another simply said, "Sorry, but we don't owe you a damn thing."

9.

THAT APRIL, MEDIUM announced that it was shutting down the publications Siobhan, my colleagues, and I had started. The financial return they were generating wasn't justifying their cost.

Although our team was offered buyouts and all but a

handful of people took them, I stayed. I was as upset as anyone else about the decision to shutter the publications; I had
helped conceive of and launch them. But I still believed in
Medium's mission of democratizing access to publishing,
and I had started working on other projects I wanted to see
through. I was also in active treatment, with annual medical
bills in the hundreds of thousands of dollars, my condition
appeared to be getting worse, not better, and we were in the
midst of a pandemic. It was a good thing I liked my job because I'm not sure I would have left Medium even if I had
wanted to.

10.

THAT SPRING, A new covid vaccine called Evusheld was introduced. Developed as a preventive measure for immunocompromised people and others at high risk for contracting a
severe case of covid, the vaccine consisted of a combination
of two monoclonal antibodies called tixagevimab and cil-
gavimab designed for preventive, as opposed to therapeutic,
purposes.

When I asked Dr. Gruenstein about the shot at one of my
weekly appointments, he suggested that I get it but told me
that he wasn't able to provide it. With demand high and supply limited, only a small number of hospitals and doctors'
offices had access to the vaccine. Because the Evusheld rollout, not unlike the rollout of other covid vaccines, was anything but well coordinated, it took me days to identify a
facility where I could receive the shot and weeks to get an
appointment.

I was originally scheduled to get the first of the two required doses in late April, but moments before receiving the
jab, after the nurse had asked me all of the requisite screen-

ing questions—or so I thought—I said to her, "Just out of an abundance of caution, can I ask you a question?"

"Of course," she said.

"I had a covid booster about a week ago. That's not an issue with Evusheld, is it?"

It turned out it was. Evusheld can reduce your body's response to the covid vaccine, rendering it, ironically, less effective.

I wound up getting my first Evusheld shot a few weeks later, on May 16, 2022. That November, I got my second dose. Two months after that, in January 2023, the FDA withdrew its approval for Evusheld. The vaccine had proven ineffective against the new variants of covid.

11.

A FEW WEEKS after I got my first Evusheld shot, Didi went to a party one night. It was held at an indoor space in Midtown, and there were twenty-five or thirty people there, some masked, some not. Several days later, she received an email from the host informing everyone who had been there that a number of attendees had contracted covid.

The next day, when Didi woke up, her throat was sore. She took a covid test, and it was positive.

Frankly, Didi was more concerned about me than she was about herself. She had been vaccinated and boosted, and most healthy people who fit that description were not getting severe cases of covid. Oscar was also fully vaccinated. Because vaccinated children seemed to be even less likely to become seriously ill than vaccinated adults, Didi and I weren't overly concerned about him, either.

I was a different story. Although I was fully vaccinated and boosted myself, and presumably even more protected by the

Evusheld, I was still considered high risk because of my weakened immune system.

Didi and I talked it over. For years, her mother has owned a small apartment near Lincoln Center. Should Didi go there? Should I? Should one of us check into a hotel?

After an hour or two of going back and forth, we decided to stay in our apartment. With A.J. away at college, her room was available. Didi would quarantine there, and Oscar and I would avoid being in the same room with her as much as possible. She would use the kids' bathroom, and Oscar and I would use the one Didi and I normally use. When Didi touched the refrigerator or kitchen sink, she wiped them down with disinfecting wipes. Anytime she left A.J.'s room, she wore a mask, and so did we. It is a strange reality that simple one-dollar masks and five-cent wipes probably did as much to keep me alive as advanced multimillion-dollar medical technologies did.

The arrangement worked. Didi went somewhat stir-crazy from living almost entirely in one room for the nine days it took for her to stop testing positive, but thankfully, she never became seriously ill, and Oscar and I did not contract covid.

A.J., for her part, seemed to be proof of the theory that some people have a natural immunity to the disease. She had been exposed to the virus numerous times through roommates, friends, and classmates and still hadn't contracted it. When she came home from college for vacations, she would test for covid as a precaution, and I would wear a mask and keep my distance from her for a few days, but after a while, we started to joke that none of that was necessary. A.J. could lick a New York City subway pole and not get covid.

A month or so after Didi got sick, on the day before Oscar was supposed to go to summer camp, he said he didn't feel well. He took a covid test, and it was positive. He, Didi, and

I essentially repeated the routine we had used when Didi was sick, in this case with Oscar quarantining in his room. He got better in a matter of days and went off to camp. Who doesn't envy the immune system of a fourteen-year-old?

We were more than two years into the pandemic. Improbably enough, despite my own weak defenses, I had still not gotten covid.

12.

WITH THE PANDEMIC ebbing, my vaccinations fully up to date, and my IgG infusions having improved my immune system function to some degree, I had begun traveling again. I was still avoiding crowded indoor spaces and wearing a mask in public places, and I was especially careful in airports and on airplanes. But Didi, Oscar, and I had flown to Ohio to visit A.J. at college, and I had gone on several fishing trips. If anything, I felt safer on the water than I did at home. On the water, I could take off my mask and breathe.

That July, I went to Idaho to fish with Tim. On the second day of my trip, less than an hour after we put our boat into the water, I started to feel dizzy and weak. I tried to shake it off, but before long, I was lying in the bottom of the boat. I could barely lift my head. Tim rowed us straight to the take-out and drove me back to the lodge where I was staying. I didn't have covid symptoms—no coughing or sneezing, no difficulty breathing, no fever—but just to be sure, I took a covid test. It was negative. I ate some soup, went straight to bed, and slept for more than eleven hours.

The next morning, I felt better and tried to rationalize the episode. Maybe I had picked up a twenty-four-hour bug. Maybe it was the altitude. Maybe I was dehydrated. But none of it really added up. I didn't seem to have any kind of virus. Altitude had never bothered me before. I had drunk plenty of water. What I felt was something I had never quite felt before. I suspected my illness was getting worse again. Whatever it was, it was the first time I had ever felt sick while fishing. The river was the last place in my life my disease hadn't touched. Now I feared that refuge was gone.

13.

AFTER I GOT home from Idaho, I got a tattoo.

Generally speaking, I don't have positive associations with the art form. Jews were tattooed by the Nazis during the Holocaust, and I had been tattooed for radiation therapy four times. Nevertheless, I knew I wanted a tattoo, and I knew exactly what I wanted it to be.

On a hot, humid August afternoon, I made an appointment at a shop near my apartment in Greenwich Village. What I came home with was the letters A and O, for A.J. and Oscar, etched in basic blue, maybe a half-inch tall, in a simple sans serif font, on the inside of my left biceps.

My single biggest fear about my illness has always been leaving my children without a father. The tattoo felt like a hedge against that.

14.

THAT FALL, I got covid. There was no clear cause. I hadn't done anything different. But thanks to my turbocharged vaccination regimen and IgG infusions, as well as a course of Paxlovid, the antiviral drug recommended for people at high risk for a serious case of the disease, I had only a mild case. I felt tired and a little weak, and my throat was scratchy, but that was about it.

The worst part was the so-called Paxlovid rebound. Almost immediately after I began taking the drug, I felt much better. But several days later, I backslid. Because of my compromised immune status—although my IgG treatment had improved my defenses, it hadn't entirely fixed them—twenty-one days passed before I stopped testing positive.

15.

THE FOLLOWING SPRING, with my disease markers getting worse, Dr. Richardson decided to extend my Darzalex and Kyprolis regimen and add back Revlimid, as well. The two drugs alone weren't working sufficiently. He explained that although Revlimid had stopped working for me previously, using a drug in combination with others sometimes produces different results. I restarted the Revlimid in May. What was originally supposed to be a six-month course of Darzalex and Kyprolis had now gone on for two-plus years.

Being back on Revlimid was strange. There was a comforting familiarity to it, like being reunited with a long-lost friend, and the drug had worked for me in the past. But it brought with it all the downsides it had previously brought, plus new ones. Not long after I restarted the Revlimid, I lost some of the feeling in my feet. (Peripheral neuropathy is a known side effect of Revlimid.) If you count the lesions on my skull, cancer had officially afflicted me from head to toe.

16.

ON OCTOBER 25, 2022, Didi and I celebrated our twenty-fifth wedding anniversary. To mark the occasion, we went away for the weekend to the Berkshires in Massachusetts. Over the course of three days, we hiked woodsy trails, took a scenic drive to the summit of 3,491-foot Mount Greylock, and saw exhibitions at the MASS MoCA and Clark Art Institute. We stayed at a cozy New England inn with a giant stone fireplace. It was the nicest time we had spent together in years. We never said it out loud, but I think we both knew why. The events of the previous months had surfaced an idea: Who knows how many more anniversaries we will get?

Didi and I are not smug married people. We have stared into the abyss of our relationship numerous times. Each of us has caused the other tremendous pain. We're well aware of how difficult, even awful, marriage can be. But we are equally aware of the pleasures marriage can bring. So far, the good has outweighed the bad. Is ours a perfect love story? Far from it. But it is still a love story.

PART EIGHT

CAR-T

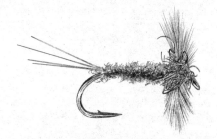

1.

THIS TIME, I didn't slip on the ice or turn around in my office chair. I bent over to load the dishwasher and felt a shot of pain in my back.

It was February 2023. Didi and I were hosting a dinner party. I knew I had been slowly coming out of remission, and the episode in the boat in Idaho had left me fearful that something new was brewing, but until then, I had been asymptomatic.

Dr. Gruenstein ordered a PET scan, but pre-authorization took more than a month. Although I had been a myeloma patient for nineteen years and was currently exhibiting classic symptoms of the disease, my insurance company kicked back the request twice, asking for additional information. Eventually, Dr. Gruenstein convinced the pre-authorization team that the procedure was necessary.

The PET scan revealed that I had not one but several new lesions: on my right hip bone, in several ribs, and in my spine.

I saw Dr. Richardson in Boston, and he decided it was time to use more powder. Because the remaining choices available to me were much more involved than anything I had done to date and would require hospitalization, he suggested that I see Dr. Jagannath in New York. Practically speaking, it didn't make sense for me to be hospitalized in Boston. "We're headed into the deep end of the pool now," he said, "aren't we, Jonathan?"

2.

ON AN INCONGRUOUSLY lovely day in March, Didi and I met with Dr. Jagannath to discuss my next treatment options.

The first thing Dr. Jagannath did was review my latest PET scans with us. I find looking inside one's own body to be simultaneously captivating and unsettling. It can be helpful to visualize exactly what's wrong with you, but there's something eerie about looking at your own innards, all the more so if they're diseased. In the same way that seeing Earth from space changed the way we think about our planet, PET scans, CT scans, and MRIs can alter the way we see ourselves. The former gave us a sense of how fragile our place in the universe is; the latter makes us see how fragile we are individually. Looking at the fire-engine red hot spots on my PET scan, I felt fragile.

My best treatment option, Dr. Jagannath explained, was going to be a cutting-edge, almost mind-blowingly futuristic type of immunotherapy called CAR T-cell therapy, or CAR-T therapy for short. It would be the most powerful form of "powder" I had used to date.

CAR-T therapy involves harvesting your T cells from your bloodstream, then sending them to a lab where a protein called a chimeric antigen receptor, or CAR, is added to the surface of the T cells (hence the acronym). The CAR protein helps the T cells recognize antigens found on the surface of specific cancer cells, in my case, myeloma cells, so the T cells can target and kill the malignant cells. The CAR-charged T cells are then infused back into your body intravenously to do their work.

The first engineered T cell with a chimeric molecule was designed in 1993 by an Israeli immunologist named Zelig Eshhar. Although early versions of the therapy proved to be ineffective, subsequent experimentation led to successful applications of the technology.

The first major breakthroughs came in 2009, when Dr. Steven Rosenberg at the National Cancer Institute successfully used CAR-T therapy to treat a lymphoma patient, and in 2010, when Dr. Carl June and Dr. David Porter from the University of Pennsylvania used the therapy to treat leukemia patients. Since then, researchers have developed CAR-T therapies that have produced unprecedented responses in patients with a variety of cancers, some of them advanced.

The technology appears to be especially effective in treating blood cancers. The particular CAR-T treatment Dr. Jagannath had in mind, a product known generically as cilta-cel (short for ciltacabtagene autoleucel) and marketed under the brand name Carvykti, was approved for use in multiple myeloma patients in February 2022, just one year and one month prior to my visit to Dr. Jagannath's office.

Although a stem cell transplant and several other therapies were still possibilities, the extraordinary promise CAR-T therapy was showing made it the clear choice for me, Dr. Jagannath said. CAR-T therapy is also a so-called one-and-done therapy; it requires little ongoing maintenance, he explained. If it worked, I could go back to living a relatively normal life, at least for a time. No pill box with M T W T F S S written on it. No passing out at concerts, diarrhea, or sleepless nights. No epic bouts of hiccups. No monthly flights to Boston. No oncological BarcaLoungers. No cancer commuting.

One of Dr. Jagannath's CAR-T therapy patients, he made a point of saying, was coming up on five years cancer free. Moreover, she was older than I was and had been sicker than I was when she had begun her treatment. Naturally, there were caveats. CAR-T therapy, he noted, is by no means 100 percent effective; it requires months of preparation, some of it complex and unpleasant, and it has a number of potentially debilitating and sometimes fatal side effects.

The scientific definition of "chimera" is a part of the body made up of tissues of diverse genetic material, but the term has two other meanings. One is an imaginary monster made up of incongruous parts. The other is an illusion, more specifically, an unrealizable dream.

3.

BECAUSE CAR-T THERAPY is an intricate, highly specialized therapy, Dr. Jagannath referred me to a CAR-T therapy specialist to manage my treatment. Didi and I had our first appointment with Dr. Shambavi Richard several weeks later.

Dr. Richard, who sports long black hair and stylish eyeglasses, balances a friendly, easygoing manner with deep professional expertise. The CAR-T therapy preparation, she explained, was indeed complex. It would include dozens of blood tests; both a bone biopsy and a bone marrow biopsy; the procedure to harvest my T cells; possibly more radiation if the bone lesions I had became problematic before I received my CAR-T therapy (it takes roughly a month after the T-cell harvest for the turbocharged cells to be manufactured); a four-day hospital stay to administer a chemotherapy regimen known as DCEP, meant to reduce the number of myeloma cells in your body to make the CAR-T treatment more effective; three days of an outpatient treatment called lymphodepletion, another form of chemotherapy that kills off your existing T cells to help the bioengineered T cells attack the myeloma cells more effectively; and the placement of a catheter in my chest that would be used to infuse the CAR-T cells, administer related medicines, and draw blood to monitor my blood counts during the two-week hospital stay the CAR-T infusion requires.

The two most serious side effects of CAR-T therapy, she told us, are cytokine release syndrome and neurotoxicity.

Cytokine release syndrome, or CRS, occurs when the body's immune system responds too aggressively to an infection (many early covid-19 patients, for reasons doctors don't fully understand, experienced CRS). In the case of CAR-T therapy, the body seems to mistake the bioengineered cells for an infection, triggering the unwelcome response. The symptoms of CRS include fever and chills ("shake and bake," as some doctors call it), fatigue, diarrhea, nausea and vomiting, headaches, cough, and low blood pressure. If not treated quickly, the condition can be fatal.

Neurotoxicity is a broad term for a set of neurological symptoms that can include headaches, confusion, delirium, slurred or incoherent speech, seizures, and cerebral edema, or swelling of the brain. It, too, can be deadly if it isn't treated immediately.

CAR-T therapy also leaves patients seriously immuno-compromised and open to infections for months and sometimes years afterward. It wipes out their immune systems so thoroughly that they eventually need to get all their childhood immunizations (mumps, measles, rubella, and so on), not to mention covid and flu shots, again. Until they get those shots, which can't be done until at least six months after CAR-T therapy, they are susceptible to all those illnesses and more. During my hospital stays, I would be allowed only a limited number of visitors, and they would all have to be masked. After I went home, I would have to live more cautiously than I had been doing, the way we all had in the early days of covid.

Didi and I had dozens of questions: Wait, how does CAR-T therapy work again? Will the T-cell harvest cause the same fire ant tingling that my stem cell harvest had caused? Will I be able to attend my niece's wedding on Cape Cod in August? In addition to being a world-class physician, Dr.

Richard is a first-rate listener. She patiently answered all our questions, told us her office would arrange the necessary appointments for us, and sent us on our way.

Didi and I took a cab home. As we made our way down Fifth Avenue, we felt strangely optimistic. Action is better than inaction. And I was going to be bionic.

4.

JUST BEFORE SHE left for college, A.J. asked me and Didi to promise that we would let her know if anything important happened with my health. After I had first told A.J. and Oscar I was sick, Didi and I had promised that we would always keep them informed about it, but A.J. wanted to be sure that we would honor our pledge. She didn't want us to feel as though we couldn't tell her something just because she was away and living on her own.

A few days after Didi and I met with Dr. Richard, I knocked on Oscar's door while he was doing his homework and told him what was going on. After explaining why I needed more treatment and what it would be, I made a point of saying my doctors were optimistic about the treatment and would be watching me carefully to make sure I got through it okay.

Oscar's main response to the news that his father was going to undergo yet another round of cancer treatment and would need to be hospitalized this time was basically that CAR-T therapy sounded cool. The idea that my T cells would be removed, altered in a lab, then put back into me to kill my cancer appealed to the science student in him. Otherwise, he seemed unfazed. It may or may not have been a pose, deliberate or otherwise, but he went back to his homework.

When I called A.J. to tell her, she expressed some concern,

but when I gave her the same spiel I had given Oscar, complete with the same reassurances, she was on board, too.

It made a certain kind of sense. I had no outward signs of illness; I didn't look, sound, or act sick. I had still never lost my hair. And kids are famously focused on themselves. That's how their brains are wired. In this circumstance, that was a good thing.

5.

I DID THE blood tests. I did the biopsies. I did the T-cell harvest (no fire ants this time; T-cell harvests generally don't trigger them the way stem cell harvests do). I didn't wind up needing radiation. In preparation for losing my hair during the two rounds of chemotherapy, I got a buzz cut. It seemed to me that losing short pieces of hair would be less traumatic than losing long strands of it. When my barber remarked that it was a dramatic choice for me, I lied and said I wanted to keep cool for the summer. On Thursday, May 11, I checked into Mount Sinai to start my four-day DCEP treatment.

DCEP is a loose acronym for "Dexamethasone, Cyclophosphamide, Etoposide, and Cisplatin," the four intravenous drugs that make up the regimen. By four o'clock that afternoon, I was ensconced in my room on the eleventh floor of the hospital and hooked up to an IV pole.

Although I was assigned to a double room, the second bed was initially unoccupied. At around 11:00 P.M., an attendant wheeled in a man who appeared to be in his late sixties or early seventies. He spoke only Spanish and was obviously seriously ill. He was moaning in pain.

Mount Sinai has interpreters whom doctors can loop into conversations with patients, but medical information can be complex, and just about every time my roommate or a member of his family attempted to communicate with the hospital staff, something, it seemed, got lost in translation.

The worst of it was a miscommunication surrounding the man's pain pump. He was obviously in severe distress, but it took three or four conversations over the course of more than a day before he fully understood how to use the pump to self-administer his medication. A hospital, let alone a cancer ward, isn't a great place to find yourself under the best of circumstances. But when you don't speak the same language as the doctors, nurses, and others who are caring for you, it is that much worse.

Kindly, the RN in charge of the ward eventually saw to it that whenever possible, the man was assigned a nurse who was fluent in Spanish. One nurse in particular hit it off with the gentleman. She called him "Papi," the affectionate term for "father." He called her "Mi querida," or "My dear." It seemed to improve things.

Because DCEP must be given continuously, I was attached to my IV around the clock. I have been hooked up to many IVs, and I can tell you that the electronic pumps used to deliver them are glitchy. The most annoying part is that the alarms the devices are equipped with, which are supposed to go off only when there is a problem with the flow of the medication, frequently go off for no reason. Every time, a nurse has to come check to be sure everything is okay, and reset the pump. When you are on a pump twenty-four hours a day, this can be maddening. It is certainly not conducive to sleeping.

After four days in the hospital, I was more than eager to go home. Physically, I felt fine. Luckily, I had tolerated the DCEP with almost no side effects. But I was exhausted and emotionally wrung out. Just after dinner on my fourth day, I was discharged.

At home, Didi, Oscar, and I took the sorts of precautions

we'd learned during the early days of the pandemic. I wore a mask, we wiped down "high-touch" surfaces frequently, and Didi and I put our toothbrushes into separate cups. To some extent, we were concerned about Didi or Oscar bringing home covid or another bug. Didi was mostly working from home and avoided going to crowded indoor places, at least not without a mask, but she sometimes went into her office, and she socialized more or less normally. And Oscar was in a large New York City public high school. He spent his days indoors among two thousand other kids. But you can worry only so much about these things, even if you have reason to be more worried about getting sick than other people do. There's only so much you can do without overly disrupting your life. You cross your fingers (or kiss the backs of your knuckles) and hope for the best.

6.

THE FIRST MORNING I was home from the hospital, after Oscar had gone to school, I sat down on the couch in our living room. Didi was at the dining room table, working on her laptop.

"You know what's nice?" I said.

From the time I had left for the hospital until that moment, I hadn't felt especially scared or upset. The events with my roommate had been unsettling, but they had been more about him than me. I could distance myself from them. Mostly, during the ninety-six hours I had been at Mount Sinai, I had just put my head down and did what I needed to do.

I started to answer my own question. What I had intended to say was "Sleeping in my own bed." But before I could finish the sentence, all the emotions I had apparently repressed over the previous four days, or maybe the previous nineteen years, came rushing to the surface.

I'm a relatively stoic person. I'm not easily overwhelmed by my problems (I'm not even particularly inclined to talk about them), and I don't complain too much (my poker whining notwithstanding). For me, stoicism isn't just a coping mechanism; it's my nature.

Well, cancer makes liars of stoics. Just as the disease attacks your body, it attacks your emotional defenses, and it doesn't stop until it strips you of them. You want to put up a fight for nineteen years? That's okay. Cancer is patient. Cancer will wait. It laughs at your perseverance. It mocks your stiff upper lip. It is amused by your courage. Eventually, it will break you. You may enter cancer as a stoic, but you will not leave as one.

I started crying. Bawling, really. A deep, primal, ugly wail. It was the first time I had cried that hard since my oldest childhood friend had written to me after I had first been diagnosed. Contrary to my stoic instincts, crying didn't make me feel weak or ashamed. It made me feel relieved. It felt as though nineteen years of weight had been lifted off my shoulders.

"I missed you guys so much," I managed to say to Didi between gasps for breath. "I am so glad to be home."

7.

AM I AFRAID of dying? Not really. Having been forced to think long and hard about the subject, I've come to terms with it. In my view, death is death. No heaven or hell. Just worm food. Nothingness. Why should I be afraid of nothing?

What I am afraid of is suffering. I have seen suffering up close, in oncologists' offices, in treatment facilities, and on cancer wards. It is decidedly scary.

During my radiation treatments, I have seen patients with skin burns so severe they look like arson victims. During my treatment sessions, I have seen a gentleman wet his pants in his chair while he was sleeping; a woman collapse on her way to the bathroom, split her head open, and bleed all over the floor; and toilets covered in splatter from diarrhea. During my hospital stays, I have seen patients who were bald, emaciated, and as pale as the hospital white blankets they were wrapped in to keep warm. I have heard moans, screams, and sounds I frankly don't know how to describe. Cancer wards have been called houses of horror. I wish I could dispute the characterization.

I'd also like to see A.J. and Oscar grow up, start their careers, get married, and have kids if they choose to. I'd like to spend my retirement with Didi, write more, fish more, play more poker, and go on more buddy trips.

I don't fear being dead. I fear not being alive.

8.

THE DCEP WAS supposed to be a lion. Physically, at least, it was a lamb. The lymphodepletion was supposed to be a lamb. It turned out to bite.

My treatments were scheduled for a Thursday, Friday, and Saturday. Sunday was left open as a rest day. Monday I would check in to the hospital for my CAR-T therapy.

Like DCEP, lymphodepletion is administered by IV but on an outpatient basis. After my first infusion, I felt okay. After the second, I felt lousy. After the third, I felt as sick as I've been from any cancer treatment I've had. I was nauseous, dizzy, and so weak that I could barely drink a glass of water or get out of bed. I had to crawl to get to the bathroom.

For better or worse, humans tend to regard a full head of

hair as a sign of good health and losing one's hair as a tell-tale sign of cancer. I've always had a good head of hair. As an adult, I've tended to wear it long on top and short on the sides, with one piece dangling over my forehead. Didi calls it my Superman curl.

Although my hair had begun to fall out somewhat during the DCEP, it now fell out completely. When I showered, the shampoo lather in my hands was flecked with countless pieces of black and gray stubble.

That was more upsetting than I'd thought it would be. My attempt to preempt that feeling by getting a buzz cut didn't really work; some things you can't prepare for. After almost twenty years, I had finally experienced perhaps the most familiar side effect of having cancer. Losing my hair was an unmistakable and undeniable sign of my illness, and it stung. The Superman curl was gone.

Even with the rest day in between, I wasn't sure I would be able to get to the hospital on Monday for my CAR-T therapy. I had visions of calling an ambulance.

People sometimes wonder if I use marijuana for nausea or pain. I smoke now and then, but for whatever reason, the drug doesn't help me. I feel all the things one normally does when one gets high, but my pain and nausea don't go away. In any event, I wasn't interested in stopgap measures. I wanted to get on with the CAR-T treatment. I wanted to be in remission.

9.

AFTER MY FINAL lymphodepletion treatment, I took a cab home from the hospital. It was Saturday, June 24, 2023, the day before the New York City Pride March, and because several major streets had been blocked off already, the traffic was gridlocked. A ride that might normally take forty-five minutes had already taken well over an hour, and I still had more than twenty blocks to go.

As we inched along Park Avenue South, a pickup truck pulled up alongside my cab. It was a red Ford F-150 with New Jersey plates. The driver and front-seat passenger were men in their early twenties, wearing tank tops and baseball caps. Bon Jovi was blasting through their open windows. If they had been characters in a movie, you would have dismissed them as too on the nose.

As one does when one is in the middle of having one's immune system wiped out in preparation for a futuristic cancer treatment, I was wearing a mask as I rode in the backseat of the cab with my window down. The driver of the pickup was now no more than a few feet from me in the lane to my right. Even before he spoke, I knew what he was going to say.

The exact quote was "Dude, lose the mask." His wingman laughed.

In my family, we like to tell a story about my father. When I was maybe five years old, all six of us—my father, my mother, my three siblings, and I—were skiing in upstate New York. It was a particularly crowded day, and there was a long line for one of the lifts.

When a group of teenagers tried to skip to the front, my father, who was a famously gentle soul but also someone who believed in rules, called them out. "Sorry, guys," he said. "We've all been waiting here a long time. You've got to go to the back of the line."

The kids ignored him.

"Guys, go to the back."

Nothing.

"Guys—"

And then: "Fuck you, old man."

That was it. Something inside my normally mild-mannered father snapped. He popped his boots out of his skis, walked over to the kids, and grabbed the leader of the pack by his coat. "Go to the back," he said. "Now!"

And to the back they went.

Back on Park Avenue South, I marshaled what strength I had at the moment and channeled my inner Gene Gluck. I got out of the cab (the traffic was stopped anyway) and stepped over to the pickup truck driver. My midstreet solilo-quy went something like this: "I'm a cancer patient, asshole. I am on my way home from a chemotherapy appointment. On Monday, I'm going into the hospital for two weeks of a treatment that could kill me. I'm wearing a mask because my immune system doesn't work. Fuck you."

In terms of the power of my performance, it didn't hurt that thanks to the DCEP and lymphodepletion, I hadn't just lost most of my hair but was also thin and ashen-looking. In fairness, the second I stepped to his window, the driver seemed to sense what was happening, and once I confirmed his suspi-cion, he seemed genuinely remorseful. "Sorry, dude," he said. "My bad."

I got back into the cab, and he and his sidekick turned right at the next cross street, I suspect to avoid having to inch along next to me any longer.

I usually don't believe in playing the cancer card. In most situations, it's too powerful a tool for the job, not to mention manipulative. But that day, I made an exception.

10.

ON MONDAY, JUNE 26, I checked in to Mount Sinai again, this time to receive my CAR-T treatment. The doctors and nurses explained to me and Didi that the infusion itself would be painless and take only half an hour or so.

After that, they would carefully monitor me—at first every fifteen minutes, then every half an hour, then every hour, and several times a day after that—for symptoms of CRS and neurotoxicity for the duration of my two-week hospital stay. (While CRS and neurotoxicity can happen weeks or even months after the CAR-T treatment is administered, they most commonly occur in the first two weeks.)

The CRS monitoring would involve blood tests and temperature and blood pressure checks. The neurotoxicity screening would entail asking me if I knew my name, what day it was, what city I was in, and so on, and handwriting tests to track my motor skills.

As we had been told before, I would be allowed only a limited number of visitors, and everyone was required to wear a mask. I came equipped with two novels, three books of crossword puzzles, and my Netflix, Hulu, and Peacock subscriptions. Jen, Tina, and Andy sent me a picture of the four of us from a family wedding to keep by my bedside.

I planned to work while I was in the hospital. Dr. Richard supported that. It would help keep my mind off of things, she said. To keep Zoom meetings from being creepy, I would either do them camera off or customize my background to something other than a hospital room.

When the time came, one of the nurses wheeled in an IV pole with the bag containing my CAR-T cells. The fluid in the bag was colorless and generally unremarkable, like so much water. I remember wondering how something so extraordinary could look so plain.

Then the nurse took the plastic line running from the bag and attached it to the catheter that had been placed in my chest earlier in the day. I watched the first few drops dangle from the valve at the bottom of the IV bag, then break loose and travel down the line into my veins.

Didi was sitting next to my bed. "Okay, cells," she said. "Work."

11.

FOR THE FIRST few days of my hospital stay, I felt fine. Not that I was having the time of my life or anything. The temperature checks, blood pressure checks, blood draws, and cognitive function tests were incessant.

"Are you in any pain?"

"No."

"I'm going to take your blood pressure now."

"Okay."

"And now your temperature."

"Sure."

And so on.

I've been stuck with needles thousands of times. I'm used to it. But being awakened every night at midnight and 3:00 A.M. to get jabbed was new to me.

Showering was a catch-22. Due to the catheter, I wasn't allowed to take a standard shower because I could develop an infection, but because of my compromised immunity, I needed to keep my skin clean to avoid infections. The prescribed solution was a special kind of disinfecting wipe that is safe to use on your skin. I can report that the wipes are a poor substitute for a shower.

For the cognitive tests, one of the doctors or nurses would ask me to write "my sentence," something they'd had me write on the first day as a baseline so they could monitor my fine motor skills. My sentence was "Today I ate breakfast, watched TV, read a book, and took a walk down the hall-way." Shakespeare!

Then would come a series of questions.

"What's your name?"

"Jonathan Gluck."

"Where are you?"

"Mount Sinai Hospital."

"In what city?"

"New York."

"How old are you?"

"Fifty-eight."

"What is that?" (Pointing to the television.)

"A television."

And so on.

Finally, they would ask me to raise my right hand, touch my finger to my nose, or some other such thing.

On the third or fourth day, when one of the nurses asked me to raise my hand, I didn't immediately do so.

She paused. "Are you okay, Jonathan?" she asked.

"You didn't say, 'Simon says.'"

For the record, she laughed.

Boredom was another issue. To pass the time, I binge-watched season two of *The Bear* (excellent). I read two books written by former *New York* magazine colleagues (*Bad Summer People,* by Emma Rosenblum, and *The Eden Test,* by Adam Sternbergh, delightfully wicked and terrifying, respectively). I finished three compilations of *New York Times* crossword puzzles (my crossword game was never stronger). And I watched literally every minute of the Tour de France, more than eighty hours of televised bicycle racing (check out Jonas Vingegaard's thrilling stage-16 time trial win, in which he deals a decisive blow to longtime rival Tadej Pogačar, on

YouTube). Because watching sports on TV has always been a kind of Prozac for me, I threw in a few dozen Wimbledon matches (delighted for Carlos Alcaraz, sad for Ons Jabeur), the women's U.S. Open golf tournament (congratulations to first-time major winner Allisen Corpuz), and a nightly dose of Yankees and Mets games (all equally and pleasantly boring). Regarding the question of whether I watched a cornhole tournament on ESPN, I plead the Fifth (go, Jamie Graham!).

If you are sensing a theme of escapism, you are not wrong. During my hospital stay for my DCEP treatment, I had read *Endurance: Shackleton's Incredible Voyage*, Alfred Lansing's account of Ernest Shackleton's ill-fated expedition. I thought the epic story of survival might inspire me (at least I wasn't stranded on an Antarctic ice floe eating seal blubber to survive), and to some extent it did. But it was also maybe a little too intense. My own saga, I decided, was harrowing enough.

I will spare you my complaints about hospital food. Actually, I won't. But I will limit them to the coffee. The coffee was horrible. Ghastly. Arguably evil. I hesitate to dignify it by calling it coffee. It was instant Nescafé, the kind done up in those skinny little packets to make them look European, dumped into a Styrofoam cupful of lukewarm water. You know the little puddles that form on the side of the road after a rainstorm, the ones with the rainbow-colored oil slicks on their surface? The coffee didn't taste like that; it tasted worse. Have you ever forgotten to change the water filter under your kitchen sink for three years, until the filter is so saturated with dirt and bacteria it could qualify as a Superfund site? Imagine wringing out that filter and drinking the byproduct. Then account for the fact that the coffee tasted ten times as bad.

On day four, I began sneaking down to the Starbucks in the hospital lobby, despite the infection risk, to get my caffeine fix. In other words, the hospital coffee was so bad that I risked my life not to drink it.

On the bright side, because I was now severely immunocompromised, I was assigned a single room. That meant I had many hours to myself. Didi has confided that she sometimes likes to go on business trips because staying in a hotel room by herself offers her a rare escape from the demands of me, the kids, the cats, and everything else. It's precious alone time. That made more sense to me than ever.

12.

MUCH OF MY time in the hospital was spent waiting for the other shoe to drop. I was told that the most likely time for cytokine release syndrome to develop, if it was going to, would be on day seven or eight after I received my CAR-T cells.

As it happened, I was on my laptop, playing in my virtual poker game, when one of the nurses came in to do a check-in. After she took my temperature, she asked me if I felt warm. I was so immersed in the card game that I hadn't noticed. But yes, I told her. Now that she mentioned it, I did feel warm.

My fever was 100.1 degrees, not enough to trigger treatment but enough to warrant closer monitoring. My checkins, which had been reduced to every three hours, were bumped back up to every thirty minutes. Luckily, my temperature never rose any higher, and after a day and a half, it returned to normal. My blood work during that period showed that the markers for CRS spiked mildly, then receded.

When Dr. Richard came to my room during rounds on day ten, she told me it looked as though I had dodged the CRS bullet. Before I could ask, she said, "No, that does not mean the CAR-T isn't working."

You have to love a doctor who assuages your fears before you can even express them.

13.

FOR YEARS, THE only way to obtain the results of medical tests was by speaking to your doctor. Either they would call you or you would call them. That could certainly be fraught. Your doctor might call at an inopportune moment, and getting results can be nerve-wracking no matter how they're delivered. Then came patient portals.

By allowing people to access their medical test results directly, portals have rewired the transactions. Signing up for a portal isn't mandatory, nor is allowing automated notifications. But doctors' offices and hospitals push people to use the portals, and as is the case with so many digital innovations, it's almost impossible to resist using them and activating the alerts.

These are more than just another distraction; they're a distraction that may have to do with your fundamental well-being or possibly even your life. If you think it's hard to resist opening the Facebook app when you see the little red circle with a number inside it, try ignoring the notice that your biopsy results are in.

That's just one problem. Medical test results are often complicated. Even if you're well versed in your disease, terminology can be hard to understand ("CMV DNA PCR, QUANT," "fibrin degrad-dimer," and "TSH w/free T4 reflex" were a few head-scratchers from my CAR-T cell stay alone). Trying to interpret results without a doctor can lead to confusion, misunderstandings, and unnecessary worry.

If your treatment is complex, you can get dozens of results in a day. Seeing all of the pings and reading all the lab tests can be overwhelming.

If you choose not to use the portals, days may pass before you get your results. If you choose not to allow the notifications, you may miss an important message.

Every now and then, I don't want to know a result when my phone pings. Maybe I've got a family vacation coming up and I don't want to know if something is wrong until after I get back. Maybe I have other stresses in my life and I'm not prepared to take on more bad news. In those instances, I'll wait for a time—an hour, a day, a week—before I open the portal to learn my fate.

But those occasions are rare. Ignoring a medical portal message takes a level of willpower that's difficult to summon. What I usually do, of course, is tap.

All that said, I was happy to have access to the Mount Sinai MyChart portal while I was getting my CAR-T treatment. After every blood test, I could check to be sure that the key measures Dr. Richard had told me about, the ones I would need to meet before I could be discharged, were normal. And every time, they brought me that much closer to going home.

14.

DIDI CAME TO the hospital every day. She brought me comforting items from home (the newspaper, clean clothes, contraband chocolate, and, before I started sneaking down to Starbucks, drinkable coffee) and kept me company. She would hold Zoom meetings in the visitor's chair in my room.

A.J. and Oscar were both at sleepaway camp, she as a counselor and he as a camper, which frankly thrilled me. I didn't want them to see me in the hospital. They knew I was there and called to check in on me, but I didn't want them to take on any additional worries about me. Seeing someone hooked up to an IV in a hospital bed isn't enjoyable, particularly not when you are a twenty-year-old or a fifteen-year-old and that someone is your father.

Some oncology wards employ what's called a "movement coordinator." One of that person's jobs is to see that patients move around as much as possible to prevent blood clots, promote healing, and so on. The movement coordinator on my ward was a cheerful fortysomething gentleman I'll call Caesar. Early on in my stay, Caesar came to my room and introduced himself, and for my first few days in the hospital, he accompanied me and my IV pole on walks up and down a long hallway just off the oncology ward.

One of the more memorable sights of my days at Mount Sinai was the parade of cancer patients, each in his or her own circle of hell, shuffling along that hallway in their hospital gowns and slippers. People in far worse shape than me were out there every day doing whatever they could to speed their recovery, escape the confines of their hospital rooms, if only briefly, or just enjoy the simple pleasure of walking, an ability more than a few of us no longer took for granted. Some slogged along for an hour or more at a time; others could manage only a few minutes. Some were speed walkers, others proceeded at a pace a slug would find slow. It was a powerful testament to the human will to survive, to get up off of the mat when you get knocked down—*Rocky* but with hospital socks and pajamas.

On day four or five, feeling claustrophobic, I asked Caesar if there was any way I could go outside. After lunch, he took me down a staff-only elevator, to avoid crowds, and across the street to Central Park, where we sat on a park bench. By any conventional measure, it was foul outside, 90-plus degrees and fetid, but to me, the air and sun felt like heaven. I had changed into street clothes, shorts and a T-shirt, and to all the world, Caesar and I must have looked like just a couple of guys enjoying a friendly afternoon chat in the park.

The next morning, Didi and I somehow found ourselves on the same park bench. After that, we started covertly busting out of the joint every day. I took to calling us the Bonnie and Clyde of Mount Sinai.

15.

ONE MORNING, WHEN I was heading back to my room after getting coffee in the lobby, I came across a yellow sticky note placed next to the Up and Down buttons on an elevator.

It read: "Every day above earth is a Good Day! Xoxo."

To the person who wrote that note, I say, "Amen."

16.

DISCHARGE DAY WAS Tuesday, July 11. I had a final check-in ("Are you in any pain?"), my catheter was removed, and I was free to go. Didi had brought a bag full of makeup, nail polish, and face creams as a thank-you gift for the nursing staff. We left it with the chief nurse and headed straight for the exits, *stat*.

On our way to the elevators, I ran into a woman I'll call Barbara. Barbara was one of the hall walkers. Scratch that. She was *the* hall walker. She was out there every day, marching back and forth for an hour or longer at a clip at least triple that of any of the rest of us. She was maybe sixty-five years old and had a strong, calm air that seemed to say, "I am aware of your power, cancer. But I'm sorry, you will not defeat me."

I was obviously leaving; I had my suitcase with me. Previously, Barbara and I had chatted a few times and exchanged small talk. But at that moment, we didn't need to speak. We understood each other perfectly, almost telepathically. What each of us was saying to the other was "I'm sorry. I understand. Good luck."

17.

WHEN DIDI AND I got home, there was a package waiting for us. It was a week's worth of dinners from Katz's Delicatessen, the old-school New York eatery. To ease our transition back to civilian life, Didi's best friend, Genevieve, and her husband, Jotham, had sent us several days' worth of meals. I single-handedly ate most of the package for lunch that day. I was starved for anything that wasn't hospital food and possibly also ravenous from euphoria.

I also took a shower, a long, hot, luxurious, I-just-got-back-from-a two-week-long-camping-trip-without-running-water kind of a shower. It was rapturous.

18.

MY NIECE SAMANTHA and her fiancé, Dylan, got married on Cape Cod about a month later, and Didi and I agonized over whether we should go. We love Sam and Dylan, and we love family weddings. Yet guests were flying in from across the country and as far away as Israel, and my immune system was as weak as it had ever been. Between my low T-cell count and my wiped-out vaccinations, I basically had the disease-fighting powers of a newborn. When I asked Dr. Richard if she thought it was safe for me to attend the wedding, she didn't give me a hard no—she said she understood that people need to live their lives—but neither was she keen on the idea. We decided not to go.

The wedding was beautiful (I've seen the pictures and watched the video), but it turned out to be a minor super-spreader event, with more than a dozen people contracting covid or the flu. Chalk up another one for Dr. Richard.

19.

ONE OF THE strange things about the pandemic was that even while it threatened to kill me, it also helped me. The fact that remote work had been normalized meant that I could continue to work from home and avoid putting myself at risk of contracting covid or other infections without having to take a leave of absence from Medium or seek other accommodations. And the fact that the pandemic normalized masking meant I could continue to wear mine without feeling too self-conscious or drawing too many strange looks.

20.

IN OCTOBER, I was due for my first post–CAR-T therapy checkup. I'd been getting tested regularly to see that my immune system was rebounding, and it was, but I hadn't yet been checked to see if the therapy had worked.

I'm still not going to call it a "second birthday," but on the day I learned my scans and blood tests were clear, that I had achieved my first full remission in five years, I had a distinct feeling of being reborn. Perhaps because the CAR-T treatment had been so deep, so *cellular,* I felt as though it had transformed me in a way that none of my previous treatments had.

Some philosophers question the idea of a continuous self, arguing that what we perceive to be the connection between our past and present selves is an illusion. On that day, I had a clear sense that my current self was wholly different from any previous incarnations. I felt physically and metaphysically new.

21.

A FEW DAYS after I learned about my remission, Dr. Richard cleared me to travel, with the usual caveats about masking, avoiding crowded indoor spaces, and the like. I called my friend Tim the next morning and booked a plane ticket to Idaho.

On the first day of that trip, I caught a big, picture-worthy brown trout. The fishing was only so-so for the remainder of the week, but Tim and I caught up on our wives, kids, and the rest of our lives. I had some good meals. At night, with the windows open and mountain air cooling the room, I slept deeply and peacefully.

It was the first time I had fished in more than a year, the longest stretch I had gone without wetting a line since I'd taken up fly-fishing three decades earlier, and the first time I had traveled since I'd had my CAR-T treatment. It felt amazing but also strange. The last time I had been in Idaho was when I had gotten sick in the boat. A lot had happened since then.

On my way back to New York, sitting at the boarding gate, a quote I had come across many years earlier came back to me. It is attributed to the ancient Greek philosopher Heraclitus. "No man ever steps in the same river twice. For it is not the same river, and he is not the same man."

22.

THE NEXT STOP on my post–CAR-T Cell Therapy Freedom Tour was A.J.'s college visiting weekend. A.J. was a drama major at Kenyon and the music director of her a cappella group, the Owl Creek Singers (named for a local river). Didi, Oscar, and I flew to Ohio to see her.

Over the course of the three-day weekend, A.J. gave us a tour of the radio station where she DJ'ed; we drank fresh-pressed apple cider and listened to a local bluegrass band at the school's Fall Harvest Festival; we attended an Owl Creek Singers performance (A.J. sang a memorable solo of Sara Bareilles's "Love Song"); and we took A.J., her girlfriend, and one of her roommates out for dinner.

On Sunday morning, before Didi, Oscar, and I flew home, the four of us met at a mom-and-pop coffee shop in town. The vibe was cozy and autumnal, and once we had our drinks, we grabbed a table next to a window looking out over the campus quad.

Another of the silver linings of the pandemic was the time we were all able to spend together. At first, during lockdown, practically all the time. Then because Didi and I had wound up working mostly remotely, we had been around most days when the kids had gotten home from school. Now, however, the four of us got together only during A.J.'s school vacations and weekends like this one.

When we were all seated at the table, A.J. said, half ironically but also half sincerely, "Well, the band is back together."

"You know," I said, "I love nothing more."

23.

FOR MANY YEARS, I kept my illness in a box: There was cancer, and there was me. Separating the two was a useful mental trick. If the first of those entities wasn't integrated into the second, perhaps I could ward it off more easily. If cancer is not a part of my actual being, maybe it's more excisable. After my CAR-T therapy, that changed. The scope and seriousness of the treatment rendered the illusion no longer believable.

In college, A.J. read a play she shared with me called *Scab*, by Sheila Callaghan. In it, a character who has been struggling with her mental health for years because of her troubled childhood tells her roommate that she has no need to go home to remind herself of her sadness. "It's my skin now," she says.

Cancer is my skin now.

24.

IN THE MONTHS leading up to the twentieth anniversary of my diagnosis, a day neither Didi nor I had been at all sure we'd see, she and I talked about how we'd like to mark the occasion.

But nothing felt right to us. A party, a trip, a "meaningful" family dinner all felt phony and staged. Besides, when I imagined those scenarios, I sensed that they'd somehow make me as sad as they'd make me happy. Surviving cancer for twenty years is obviously something to be glad about, but being sick for twenty years is a weird thing to celebrate.

The week before the anniversary, I had an idea: Why not use the occasion to honor the doctors and researchers who have kept me and countless other myeloma patients alive and support their future efforts? In that spirit, we launched a Go-FundMe for myeloma research, with our family promising to match donations up to $10,000.

A.J. was away at school, but she, Didi, Oscar, and I were watching the GoFundMe ticker and texting one another as the donations came in. Friends from my childhood donated, friends from high school and college, friends from old jobs, friends of Didi's, friends of A.J.'s and Oscar's, one of the kids' childhood babysitters.

Within five hours, we had reached our $10,000 goal, and by the end of the week, 164 people had donated $20,852. Two people we know contributed another $5,000 and $500, privately, off the platform. After the matching donation Didi and I made, we raised a total of $36,962.

At one point in the group chat, A.J. wrote, "You are pretty loved," and I replied, "Genuinely humbled by all the love out there for all of the Glucks."

But Didi put it best. "People," she wrote, "are amazing."

25.

AS A SOCIETY, we tend to make saints of the sick. We impart nobility to suffering. Who knows why? Out of sympathy, I suppose.

I'm here to tell you that I'm nobody's saint. Just because I have cancer doesn't mean I can't be arrogant, apathetic, deceitful, disrespectful, greedy, impatient, judgmental, manipulative, mean, petty, rude, or selfish. I can be all of those things and worse. All of us are sinners, and all of us are saints. Illness doesn't sanctify us.

26.

ON THE MORNING of Saturday, November 4, 2023, I woke up before Didi. I was in our living room reading when she came in to say good morning. Oscar was still asleep.

Didi told me about a dream she'd had. She was in Northampton, Massachusetts, the next town over from her hometown. A crowd had gathered on the main street, and they were looking up at the streetlights. Some people, including a woman holding a baby, were perched on top of it, like birds. Didi yelled to them to be careful or they were going to fall. Sure enough, one woman lost her footing, and the crowd gasped. But on her way down, the woman somehow grabbed the pole and shimmied to safety. She walked away unhurt.

Didi and I batted around some ideas about what the dream might mean—Did she know someone who'd had a baby lately? Had she been thinking about Amherst for some reason?—but none of our theories resonated.

We started chatting about the fundraiser and checked to see if there had been new contributions overnight. Then Didi said, "By the way, Happy Anniversary of Being Alive." Until then, I hadn't registered that the day was *that* day. Then she said, "Oh, my God, the dream." Someone nearly dying but somehow improbably, almost impossibly even, surviving?

For the rest of the day, I did what I would normally do on a Saturday: I went for a walk along the Hudson River. I went grocery shopping. I talked on the phone with my mother.

Didi, Oscar, and I went out for dinner, then watched a movie on Netflix. It was all utterly unremarkable. Boring never felt so good.

The next morning, Didi and Oscar went out to run errands. Poking around the apartment, I caught a reflection of myself in our hallway mirror, and two words popped into my head: *Twenty years*.

Once again, I found myself shaking my head.

PART NINE

Reflection

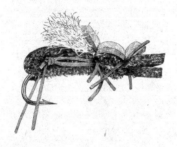

1.

I'M SOMETIMES ASKED what being sick for so long has taught me. If I had to summarize it, this is what I'd say.

You can handle more than you think you can. When I was diagnosed with cancer, I didn't think I could manage such a daunting challenge. After surviving for twenty years, I know I can.

People, most of them anyway, are good. That's especially true of doctors and nurses.

If you do work you enjoy, you are lucky.

If you have money, medical insurance, and other privileges, you are even luckier.

If you have a family and friends who love and support you, you are luckier still.

Tragedies happen. So do miracles. I didn't think I would get cancer in the first place. I did. I didn't think I could survive it. So far, anyway, I have.

If there's something you want to do, do it now.

A good relationship is worth fighting for, even if it goes bad for a time.

Love isn't always pretty. That doesn't mean it isn't love.

I will never love anything more than I love my kids.

If you know someone who is sick, lend them a hand. At the very least, tell them you're sorry about what they're going through and wish them well. It will make both of you feel better.

Say yes more than no.

Travel. Or fish. Or juggle. Or do needlepoint. It doesn't matter what you do. Do something that reliably brings you happiness.

If you're worried about something, do something, anything, to take your mind off of it. "Nature abhors a vacuum," Aristotle said. Worry loves one.

The difference between the sick and the well isn't a difference in kind. It's a difference of timing. While the well have the luxury of not thinking about death, the sick do not. The irony is that a heightened awareness of death can teach us how to live. If only the well could absorb that knowledge. If only the sick could live long enough to enjoy it.

Perhaps the biggest lesson I've learned is to accept whatever life brings my way. Sometimes the fish are biting, sometimes they're not. Sometimes the cards fall your way, sometimes they don't. Sometimes you are sick, sometimes you are well. Controlling what you can control and accepting what you can't may not be the secret of human happiness, but it's probably as close as we're going to get.

In his 2003 book *A Mathematician Plays the Stock Market,* Temple University math professor and philosopher John Allen Paulos put it this way: "Uncertainty is the only certainty there is, and knowing how to live with insecurity is the only security."

2.

NOT LONG AGO, I asked Didi how my diagnosis and illness have affected her. Physically, she said, she sometimes still gets stress-related migraines and back problems. "But I'm also better about going to my physicals, mammograms, and other basic exams," she said. "I see how much good doctoring has helped you." Mentally, she said, she still sometimes gets depressed about my diagnosis. "I also still get angry and then also still feel guilty about having those feelings, because you have it far worse than I do."

Her friends have been invaluable, she said. "I talk to them

whenever you are diagnosed or rediagnosed, but sometimes I also turn to them just to get out of being in the cancer world all the time. Like, I itch to get out."

Her mother always asks how I am, she said, but sometimes it's difficult for them to talk about my illness. "I think it's hard for us to dwell on sickness and death because we experienced so much of it together."

She said it's difficult for her to say if cancer has influenced what kind of a mother she is. "I've literally only been a mom without a husband who has cancer for seven months."

She may go overboard on prioritizing work, she said, because it pulls her into a different world and because on some level she feels the need to provide for our family if someday I can't. "Remember, this isn't my first brush with primary breadwinner loss."

Sometimes, she still feels as though she can never live up to what I want from her. "But more than that, I feel like whatever I do isn't enough because I can't take away your illness or go through the treatments for you." She said she sometimes wishes our roles were reversed. "You hate to see someone you love sick—or worse, in pain. You wish you had a magic wand to make it go away. If cancer is an exercise in uncertainty, being a caregiver is an exercise in futility."

She said she doesn't know what our marriage would have been like if I hadn't gotten sick. "At this point, I can't imagine it any other way." What she does know, she said, is that no marriage doesn't have a "thing." "If it weren't cancer, maybe one of us would have had another illness. Or changed careers. Or won the lottery. Who knows? Who cares? Cancer is our thing."

In terms of losing me, she said, her answer is similar to what she said about being a mom. "I've been married to 'cancer you' much longer than 'noncancer you.' I've sort of gone through all the stages of grief over the past twenty-plus years. I've been sad, angry, acted out . . . and ultimately come to accept that this is what it is and there is no 'cancer you' or 'healthy you.' There's just you."

As far as A.J. and Oscar go, she said, she worries less with every passing day about how they will fare if I die. "They're older now than I was when my father died. If you die because of myeloma—and as Dr. Gruenstein says, 'May you live to a hundred and get hit by a bus'—I'll tell them what I have come to believe. That we are made from our parents, so they will always be a part of us."

3.

PEOPLE OFTEN WONDER if I've changed the way I eat and exercise. The answer is that I try to take better care of myself than I did before I was diagnosed, but I haven't gone monastic. I don't eat faux orange foods anymore (much), and I try to get to the gym as often as I can. But I still use a cellphone and stand in front of the microwave and sometimes eat and drink too much or don't get off my sofa for a couple of days at a time.

Getting sick has certainly taught me the importance of good health, but I don't see the point of living if you don't enjoy your life.

To me, the question is more interesting than the answer. People want to believe that we can fend off illness with broccoli or ginseng or goji berries. When I tell them I haven't gone vegan, started taking nutritional supplements, or taken up hot yoga, some people even seem judgmental. *You have cancer and you haven't gone macrobiotic? Don't you want to live?*

I don't have anything against diet or exercise practices

that might help improve a person's health or even just make them feel good. But my cancer wasn't caused by lifestyle choices, and it's not going to be cured by them. I wish it were that simple.

At the same time, I sometimes find myself angry at people who don't take care of themselves, especially if they're doing something known to make them sick. Smokers, for example. Not because I judge them but because I feel that they're taking their health for granted. I sometimes have the urge to stop smokers on the street and tell them my story, like some kind of impromptu *Scared Straight* lecture.

And I do believe that everyone should get mammograms, colonoscopies, and other routine cancer screenings. Even with the dramatic advances in cancer treatment, early detection is critical. I don't always practice what I preach. Even after all I've been through, I sometimes put off my own surveillance tests; I'm only human. But I can't say I recommend it.

If there are five words in the English language I am sure of, they are: *You do not want cancer.*

4.

IN CASE I haven't been clear: Cancer is awful. I have been diagnosed and rediagnosed with the disease and gone into and out of remission so many times I've stopped counting. I've run a gauntlet of treatments and experienced countless unwelcome side effects. I've had enough drugs pumped into me to make Keith Richards jealous. I've spent thousands of hours in doctors' offices and hospitals and hundreds of thousands of dollars out of my own pocket on medical care, despite having good insurance. I've waited more than seven hours to see one doctor. I've spent a year and a half resolving a single billing dispute. I've logged on to and off of more provider portals than I care to remember. I've confirmed my date of birth and address. I've given my phone number in case we get disconnected. The last four digits of my Social Security number are . . .

Cancer has upended my physical and mental health, my marriage, my children, my career, and frankly, every other aspect of my life. Just as the disease metastasizes throughout the body, so does it spread through one's life. As I type this, I am fifty-nine years old chronologically, but biologically, I sometimes feel like Methuselah if Methuselah had spent more than a third of his 969 years fighting cancer.

What would I give to erase the events of November 4, 2003? What would I give never to have another marrow biopsy or PET scan or blood draw? What would I give never to have another radiation treatment or chemotherapy session or immunotherapy infusion? What would I give never to be stuck with another needle? What would I give never to see another doctor or endure another hospital stay? What would I give never to fight again with an insurance company? What would I give never to have to worry about the next recurrence of my disease? What would I give for my wife, my kids, my friends, and my family never to have to worry about me?

What would I give?

What wouldn't I give?

5.

WHY AM I alive?

I am fortunate to have tremendous love and support from a spouse, family, and friends, I can afford good healthcare, and I am a white male. Research shows that these factors all contribute to better-than-average health outcomes.

I have heredity on my side. All four of my grandparents lived into their nineties, my father lived until he was ninety, and my mother is still alive at ninety-three.

And I have been plain old lucky. As Dr. Weiner once pointed out, that slip on the ice was "an angel's kiss": It tipped me off to my cancer relatively early, before it had a chance to spread. (Did you know that *Glück* is German for "luck"?)

But in the end, I am alive because of science.

The treatments and medications I've had, developed over the centuries through the intelligence and hard work of countless men and women who have devoted their lives to finding a cure for cancer and the similarly dedicated doctors and nurses who administer cancer care—they are the reasons I am here.

6.

WHAT'S GOING TO happen to me next? When I come out of remission, another recently developed treatment called bispecific antibodies will likely be my next option. A cutting-edge type of immunotherapy treatment, bispecific antibodies are agents designed to simultaneously bind to T cells and tumor cell antigens. The idea is to turbocharge your T cells and speed tumor death at the same time—a powerful one-two punch. A stem cell transplant remains a possibility for me as well, as do a number of other older therapies I haven't yet been treated with.

There are also promising therapies in development. Dr. Richardson, for one, is working on an oral agent called mezigdomide that activates the immune system and directly kills myeloma cells—a next-generation Pomalyst, so to speak, that has shown encouraging early results for patients with very advanced disease, which is a rarity. While artificial intelligence may put me and other writers and editors out of work, it also promises to be a powerful new weapon in the fight against cancer. In addition to facilitating faster and more accurate diagnoses, AI is being used to analyze DNA to improve our understanding of the biology of cancer and to develop better and less toxic therapies for it. It can also analyze patterns in medical data with unprecedented speed to determine which drug combinations might work best to treat specific cancers.

Personalized cancer therapies are another encouraging area of research. Breakthroughs in the understanding of DNA are allowing doctors to match specific therapies to individual patients based on their unique genetic fingerprint. A patient's DNA can tell doctors which specific subtype of a cancer they have, allowing physicians to tailor treatment to that exact subtype. It can also give doctors clues as to which patients will respond best to which medicines, again paving the way for customized treatment.

Those are all exciting possibilities, but they are just that: possibilities. Unless those or other new myeloma treatments are developed in the not-too-distant future, I will eventually run out of options. Sometimes, it feels as though I'm locked in a basement that's slowly filling with water.

7.

AFTER TWO FAILED attempts and a lifetime of dreaming about it, I finally took my trip to Alaska. In June 2022, I flew to the Katmai Peninsula for a five-day fishing excursion. The trip had its hiccups—we got fogged in one day, the airline lost my luggage on my flight home—but, in all, it was spectacular. I bombed around from one virtually untouched fishing hole to the next in bush planes, saw mama grizzly bears and their cubs at a distance of no more than twenty-five feet, and caught some of the biggest fish I've caught in my life, including my first salmon on a fly.

Just before lunch on the final day, a guide, another guest, and I flew to the mouth of a stream called Margot Creek, where it empties into Naknek Lake in the shadow of the famed Brooks Range. The creek was cold and clear, the sky was a deep cobalt blue, and nine-thousand-foot summits towered above us. Before we started fishing, we set up a picnic lunch—lamb gyros on homemade pita bread, hot bison chili, and Rice Krispies Treats—and ate next to the plane.

After we were done, we waded up Margot Creek. My companions caught a handful of fish, but for the first time in three days, I was shut out. As we headed back to the plane, I decided to try my luck in one last spot.

On my first cast, I watched my fly drift downstream. For a second, nothing. Another second, still nothing. Then I felt a strike. After a short fight, I brought a fat, sixteen-inch Dolly Varden to hand. It was a gorgeous creature with spearmint-and-orange markings dappling its sides. The high alpine sun bathed it in an ethereal light. The scene was majestic, almost mystical. If the mountains or the river had up and spoken to me, I wouldn't have been surprised.

After a moment, I removed the hook from the fish's mouth, lowered it into the water, and released it. With a flick of its tail, it returned to the unknown.

Acknowledgments

Mark Adams taught me how to write a book proposal and introduced me to my literary agent, Daniel Greenberg. In addition to helping me sell this book, Daniel provided invaluable input into how to shape it.

For years, Jordan Pavlin encouraged me to pursue this project; she also offered expert guidance along the way.

As early readers, Eric Hattler, Robert Kolker, Mark Jannot, Annika Martin, Genevieve Monsma, and Adam Moss offered indispensable advice. As a final reader, Maura Fritz did the same.

Matthew Benjamin, my editor, offered brilliant editorial insight that made each iteration of this work vastly better, and did so with an unfailingly warm and sensitive touch.

David Bjerklie contributed substantial medical reporting. Lynn Anderson and Julie Tate provided meticulous copy editing and fact-checking, respectively. Mia Pulido offered critical production assistance.

Allison Applebaum, Catherine Sanderson, and Kate Sweeny helped me understand the psychological and emotional effects of cancer on patients and their caregivers.

Bill Shapiro gave me my first job in journalism. John Rasmus, Caroline Miller, Anna Wintour, Joanna Coles, and Siobhan O'Connor were also kind enough to hire me. Jeffries Blackerby, David DiBenedetto, Michael Idov, Mark Jannot, Bob Love, Emma Rosenblum, Daniel Saltzstein, Sandhya Somashekhar, Michael Steele, and Amy Virshup all published stories of mine that helped lead to this book.

More than anyone else, my high school English teacher Geoff Marchant taught me how to read and write, and love doing both.

Among the works I drew upon to write this book, none were more important than *The Emperor of All Maladies: A Biography of Cancer,* by Siddhartha Mukherjee, *Between Two Kingdoms: A Memoir of a Life Interrupted,* by Suleika Jaouad, and *Stand by Me,* by Allison Applebaum. Rebecca Skloot's *The Immortal Life of Henrietta Lacks,* Elizabeth Gilbert's *Eat, Pray, Love: One Woman's Search for Everything Across Italy, India and Indonesia,* and Joan Didion's *The Year of Magical Thinking* were also influences.

David DiBenedetto, Ryan D'Agostino, Eric Hattler, Mark Jannot, Robert Kolker, Randy Parker, Ted Putala, Bill Shapiro, Tim Warren, David Willey, Jeffrey Wright, and David Ziskin are the very definition of friends. I am forever grateful for their love, kindness, and support.

There are no words powerful enough to express my gratitude to Dr. Lon Weiner, Dr. Patrick Boland, Dr. Steven Gruenstein, Dr. Paul Richardson, Dr. Sundar Jagannath, Dr. Shambavi Richard, Dr. Tarek Mouhieddine, and the countless other physicians, medical researchers, nurses, and other healthcare practitioners who have done nothing less than save my life.

Dr. Barbara Gol helped me achieve levels of peace and happiness I could not have achieved without her. Hilary Weinger did the same for both me and Didi.

Patty Rodriguez and Danielle Costanza didn't just help me and Didi raise our family; they *are* family.

Phil Taylor, Danny Conroy, and Heidi Munyer helped keep me fit and moving.

My parents, Gene and Betsy Gluck, taught me everything important I ever needed to know.

My sisters, Jennifer Gluck and Tina Henderson, and my brother, Andy Gluck, along with their spouses, children, and children's families, have been unshakable pillars of love and support, as have Didi's mother, Estela Olevsky, and her partner, George Greenstein.

My wife, Didi, and my children, A.J. and Oscar, are everything to me.

Notes

Part One: The Slip

9   **At the time I learned:** Here and elsewhere, the source I used for multiple myeloma and other cancer survival rates is "Cancer Stat Facts: Myeloma," National Cancer Institute, https://seer.cancer.gov /statfacts/html/mulmy.html.

10   **According to a National Health Council report:** "About Chronic Diseases," National Health Council, https://nationalhealthcouncil.org /wp-content/uploads/2019/12/NHC_Files/Pdf_Files/AboutChronic Disease.pdf.

Part Two: Diagnosis

15   **"This isn't possible":** Portions of this book pertaining to the first three and a half years following my diagnosis are adapted from my essay "The Radioactive Dad," *New York,* May 18, 2007, https:// nymag.com/news/features/2007/cancer/32122/.

19   **Despite claims to the contrary:** Joanna Walters, "Former EPA Head Admits She Was Wrong to Tell New Yorkers Post-9/11 Air Was Safe," *Guardian,* September 10, 2016, https://www.theguardian.com/us -news/2016/sep/10/epa-head-wrong-911-air-safe-new-york-christine -todd-whitman.

19   **the air, as we now know:** Julia Preston, "Public Misled on Air Quality After 9/11 Attack, Judge Says," *New York Times,* February 3, 2006, https://www.nytimes.com/2006/02/03/nyregion/public-misled-on-air -quality-after-911-attack-judge-says.html.

22   **As of 2023:** "Health Insurance Coverage: Early Release of Estimates

from the National Health Interview Survey, 2023," National Center for Health Statistics report, June 2024, https://www.cdc.gov/nchs/data/nhis/earlyrelease/insur202406.pdf.

22 **Uninsured people are less likely:** J. Michael McWilliams, "Health Consequences of Uninsurance Among Adults in the United States: Recent Evidence and Implications," *Milbank Quarterly* 87, no. 2 (June 2009): 443–94, https://www.ncbi.nlm.nih.gov/pmc/articles/PMC2881446/.

22 **More than 65 percent:** David U. Himmelstein et al., "Medical Bankruptcy: Still Common Despite the Affordable Care Act," *American Journal of Public Health* 109, no. 3 (March 2019): 431–33, https://www.ncbi.nlm.nih.gov/pmc/articles/PMC6366487/.

25 **In the years since:** Here and elsewhere, the information about the history, biology, and treatment of multiple myeloma came primarily from the following sources: "Plasma Cell Neoplasms (Including Multiple Myeloma) Treatment (PDQ)—Patient Version," National Cancer Institute, https://www.cancer.gov/types/myeloma/patient/myeloma-treatment-pdq#_162; "Understanding Multiple Myeloma," Multiple Myeloma Research Foundation, https://themmrf.org/multiple-myeloma; "Multiple Myeloma Treatment Overview," Multiple Myeloma Research Foundation, 2021, https://themmrf.org/wp-content/uploads/2023/05/Treatment-Overview_Booklet_2022_012022-1.pdf; "Treatments for Multiple Myeloma," Multiple Myeloma Research Foundation, https://themmrf.org/diagnosis-and-treatment/treatment-options/. My personal physicians provided additional information.

34 **By some estimates:** Linda T. Kohn, Janet M. Corrigan, and Molla S. Donaldson, eds., *To Err Is Human: Building a Safer Health System* (Washington, DC: National Academies Press, 2000), https://pubmed.ncbi.nlm.nih.gov/25077248/.

34 **with some reports putting that number:** Vanessa McMains, "Johns Hopkins Study Suggests Medical Errors Are Third-Leading Cause of Death in U.S.," Johns Hopkins University, May 3, 2016, https://hub.jhu.edu/2016/05/03/medical-errors-third-leading-cause-of-death/.

43 **Radiation therapy dates back:** "History of Cancer Treatments: Radiation Therapy," American Cancer Society, https://www.cancer.org/cancer/understanding-cancer/history-of-cancer/cancer-treatment-radiation.html; Hyun Do Huh and Seonghoon Kim, "History of Ra-

diation Therapy Technology," *Progress in Medical Physics* 31, no. 3 (2020): 124–34, https://www.progmedphys.org/journal/view.html?doi=10.14316/pmp.2020.31.3.124.

Part Three: Limbo

52 **For a time, I took Vioxx:** *Vioxx: The Downfall of a Drug,* National Public Radio, various episodes, https://www.npr.org/series/5033105/vioxx-the-downfall-of-a-drug.

63 **The late Dr. Herbert Benson:** Scott Edwards, "Fly-Fishing and the Brain," *On the Brain,* series, Harvard Medical School, Summer 2015, https://hms.harvard.edu/news-events/publications-archive/brain/fly-fishing-brain.

64 **Similar programs exist:** See, e.g., "About Us," Reel Recovery, https://reelrecovery.org, and Casting for Recovery, https://castingforrecovery.org.

68 **In one study Sweeny led:** Kate Sweeny and Sara E. Andrews, "Mapping Individual Differences in the Experience of a Waiting Period," *Journal of Personality and Social Psychology* 106, no. 6 (June 2014): 1015–30, https://www.katesweeny.com/uploads/2/6/9/4/26944848/sweeny__andrews_2014_jpsp.pdf.

68 **In 2019, she and fellow researchers:** Kyla Rankin, Lisa C. Walsh, and Kate Sweeny, "A Better Distraction: Exploring the Benefits of Flow During Uncertain Waiting Periods," *Emotion* 19, no. 5 (August 2019): 818–28, https://www.katesweeny.com/uploads/2/6/9/4/26944848/rankin_walsh___sweeny_2018__emotion_.pdf.

69 **In 2020, Sweeny and other researchers:** Kate Sweeny et al., "Flow in the Time of COVID-19: Findings from China," *PLOS ONE,* November 11, 2020, https://journals.plos.org/plosone/article?id=10.1371/journal.pone.0242043.

70 **In one study:** Kyla Rankin, Dakota Le, and Kate Sweeny, "Preemptively Finding Benefit in a Breast Cancer Diagnosis," *Psychology & Health* 35, no. 5 (May 2020): 613–28.

72 **In an attempt:** Catherine A. Sanderson, "The Psychology of Understanding and Managing Uncertainty," *Psychology Today,* September 21, 2021, https://www.psychologytoday.com/us/blog/norms-matter/202109/the-psychology-understanding-and-managing-uncertainty.

73 **When we spoke:** David A. Sbarra and Paul J. Nietert, "Divorce and Death: Forty Years of the Charleston Heart Study," *Psychological Sci-*

ence 20, no. 1 (January 2009): 107–13, https://www.ncbi.nlm.nih.gov
/pmc/articles/PMC2977944/.

Part Four: Recurrence

104 **When I was a kid:** Some of the material about my father is adapted
from my essay "The Father's Day Fishing Trip I'll Never Forget," Medium, June 19, 2020, https://humanparts.medium.com/the-fathers
-day-fishing-trip-i-ll-never-forget-3644a64a271d.

Part Five: RVD

117 **The history of cancer:** The sources I consulted on the history of cancer and cancer treatment include "The History of Cancer," American
Cancer Society, https://www.cancer.org/cancer/understanding-cancer
/history-of-cancer.html; Siddhartha Mukherjee, *The Emperor of All
Maladies: A Biography of Cancer* (New York: Scribner, 2010); Jennet
Conant, "How a WWII Disaster—and Cover-up—Led to a Cancer
Treatment Breakthrough," History, August 12, 2020, https://www
.history.com/news/wwii-disaster-bari-mustard-gas; Edward J. Odes et
al., "Earliest Hominin Cancer: 1.7-Million-Year-Old Osteosarcoma
from Swartkrans Cave, South Africa," *South African Journal of Science* 112, no. 7/8 (July–August 2016), https://sajs.co.za/article/view
/3566/4505; Jordan Pearson, "Ancient Skull with Brain Cancer Pre-
serves Clues to Egyptian Medicine," *New York Times*, May 29, 2024,
https://www.nytimes.com/2024/05/29/science/brain-cancer-ancient
-egypt-skull.html; Luca Falzone, Salvatore Salomone, and Massimo
Libra, "Evolution of Cancer Pharmacological Treatments at the Turn
of the Third Millennium," *Frontiers in Pharmacology* 9 (November 12, 2018), https://www.frontiersin.org/journals/pharmacology
/articles/10.3389/fphar.2018.01300/full; "What Are the Pillars of
Cancer Treatment?," Vial, https://vial.com/blog/articles/what-are-the
-pillars-of-cancer-treatment/?utm_source=organic; Robert D. Carl-
son, John C. Flickinger, Jr., and Adam E. Snook, "Talkin' Toxins:
From Coley's to Modern Cancer Immunotherapy," *Toxins* 12, no. 4
(April 2020): 241, https://www.mdpi.com/2072-6651/12/4/241.

126 **Dr. Judah Folkman:** Judah Folkman, "Tumor Angiogenesis: Thera-
peutic Implications," *New England Journal of Medicine* 285, no. 21
(November 18, 1971): 1182–86, https://www.nejm.org/doi/abs/10.1056
/NEJM197111182852108.

128 **A 2021 article:** Carmen-Maria Rusz et al., "Off-Label Medication: From a Simple Concept to Complex Practical Aspects," *International Journal of Environmental Research and Public Health* 18, no. 19 (October 4, 2021): 10447, https://www.ncbi.nlm.nih.gov/pmc/articles/PMC8508135 /#B63-ijerph-18-10447; James H. Stoeckle et al., "The Evolving Role and Utility of Off-Label Drug Use in Multiple Myeloma," *Exploration of Targeted Anti-tumor Therapy* 2, no. 4 (August 2021): 355–73, https:// www.explorationpub.com/Journals/etat/Article/100250.

128 **In "The Evolving Role":** Stoeckle et al., "The Evolving Role and Utility of Off-Label Drug Use in Multiple Myeloma."

130 **In 2010:** Paul G. Richardson et al., "Lenalidomide, Bortezomib, and Dexamethasone Combination Therapy in Patients with Newly Diagnosed Multiple Myeloma," *Blood* 116, no. 5 (August 2010), https:// ashpublications.org/blood/article/116/5/679/107744/Lenalidomide -bortezomib-and-dexamethasone.

145 **Disability claims are among:** "EEOC Releases Two Litigation Program Updates," U.S. Equal Employment Opportunity Commission, March 27, 2024, https://www.eeoc.gov/newsroom/eeoc-releases-two -litigation-program-updates.

149 **Research on the subject:** Kelly L. Wierenga, Rebecca H. Lehto, and Barbara Given, "Emotion Regulation in Chronic Disease Populations: An Integrative Review," *Research and Theory for Nursing Practice* 31, no. 3 (August 2017): 247–71, https://www.ncbi.nlm.nih.gov/pmc /articles/PMC5992894/.

155 **But a study published in 2023:** Alexandros Katsiferis, "Sex Differences in Health Care Expenditures and Mortality After Spousal Bereavement: A Register-Based Danish Cohort Study," *PLOS ONE,* March 22, 2023, https://journals.plos.org/plosone/article?id=10.1371/journal.pone .0282892.

162 **I asked my friend:** The material about fly-fishing in the Bahamas is adapted from my article "The Best Place in the World for Bonefishing Is No Picnic," Bloomberg, August 31, 2015, https://www.bloomberg .com/news/features/2015-08-31/the-best-place-in-the-world-for -bonefishing-is-no-picnic?embedded-checkout=true.

183 **Patagonia is one of the world's:** The material about fly-fishing in Patagonia is adapted from my article "Angling for a Whopper in the Fly-Fishing Paradise of Patagonia," *New York Times,* March 6, 2019, https://www.nytimes.com/2019/03/06/travel/chile-patagonia-fly -fishing.html.

Part Six: Clinical Trial

208   **Instead of jetting off:** The material about fly casting in the street in front of my apartment is adapted from my essay "Fly Casting on City Streets Is Weird. That's Why I Love It," *New York Times Magazine,* August 5, 2020, https://www.nytimes.com/2020/08/05/magazine/fly -casting-on-city-streets-is-weird-thats-why-i-love-it.html.

Part Seven: Immunotherapy

222   **That January, I wrote:** "This Is a Dangerous Time in the Pandemic for People like Me. Don't Forget Us," *Washington Post,* January 17, 2022, https://www.washingtonpost.com/outlook/2022/01/17/immuno compromised-pandemic-omicron.

Part Nine: Reflection

273   **There are also promising therapies:** Paul G. Richardson et al., "Mezigdomide Plus Dexamethasone in Relapsed and Refractory Multiple Myeloma," *New England Journal of Medicine* 389, no. 11 (August 30, 2023): 1009–22, https://www.nejm.org/doi/full/10.1056 /NEJMoa2303194.

274   **In June 2022:** A portion of the material about Alaska is adapted from my article "A Fly Fisherman's Alaskan Adventure," *Garden & Gun,* August–September 2023, https://gardenandgun.com/feature /a-fly-fishermans-alaskan-adventure/.

About the Author

JONATHAN GLUCK is a writer and an editor whose work has appeared in *The New York Times* and *The Washington Post*. He was deputy editor of *New York* magazine for ten years, after which he worked as managing editor of *Vogue*. His work has been recognized with multiple National Magazine Awards.

About the Type

THIS BOOK was set in Sabon, a typeface designed by the well-known German typographer Jan Tschichold (1902–74). Sabon's design is based upon the original letter forms of sixteenth-century French type designer Claude Garamond and was created specifically to be used for three sources: foundry type for hand composition, Linotype, and Monotype. Tschichold named his typeface for the famous Frankfurt typefounder Jacques Sabon (c. 1520–80).